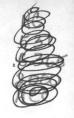

OVERCOMING ANXIETY, PANIC, AND DEPRESSION

New Ways To Regain Your Confidence

James Gardner, M.D.   Arthur H. Bell, Ph.D.

**CAREER
PRESS**
Franklin Lakes, NJ

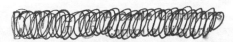

Overcoming Anxiety, Panic, and Depression
Cover design by Design Solutions
Printed in the U.S.A. by Book-mart Press

To order this title, please call toll-free 1-800-CAREER-1 (NJ and Canada: 201-848-0310) to order using VISA or MasterCard, or for further information on books from Career Press.

The Career Press, Inc., 3 Tice Road, PO Box 687, Franklin Lakes, NJ 07417

Please Note:

This book contains information that the authors believe to be correct. However, no recommendation for any individual's treatment, therapy, or medical care is intended, expressed, or implied. No reader should act on the basis of any printed medical information, including the contents of this book, without consultation with a health professional.

Library of Congress Cataloging-in-Publication Data
Gardner, James, 1959-
     Overcoming anxiety, panic, and depression : new ways to regain your confidence / by James Gardner and Art Bell.
          p. cm.
     Includes index.
     ISBN 1-56414-435-6 (paper)
     1. Anxiety—Popular works. 2. Panic disorders—Popular works.
     3. Depression, Mental—Popular works. I. Bell, Arthur H. (Arthur Henry),
1946-   II. Title.

RC531.G365 1999
616.85'223—dc21

99-05268

Dedication

For James C. Gardner, M.D.

This book is dedicated with gratitude and love to my wife, Patty, who provides the organized and comfortable environment that makes my work and writing possible. Her friendship, humor, faith and selflessness are always a source of great encouragement and inspiration.

For Arthur H. Bell, Ph.D.

I dedicate my work here with love to my wife, Dayle, and to my children Art, Lauren, and Madeleine. They are in every sense my inspiration.

Acknowledgments

For James C. Gardner, MD:

As a General Physician, I drew on the advice, teaching, and counsel of many in preparing this book. Of my many mentors and teachers, I would especially like to thank Tanya Atagi, M.D., James Puffer, M.D., Martin Pope, M.D., David Busch, M.D., Bob Lukas, M.D., Marvin Ginsburg, M.D., James Ungar, M.D., Harit Rana, M.D., David Tully-Smith, M.D., Matthew Cushing, M.D., Michael Gitlin, M.D., and Troy L. Thompson II, M.D.

Those who were generous with their time and advice on specific matters pertaining to this book include Javald I. Sheikh, M.D., William Barton, Ph.D., MFCC, John H. Greist, M.D., David Christianson, Stephen M. Stahl, M.D., Ph.D., Timothy West, Ph.D., Barbara Stockwell, Barbara Rose Billings, Ph.D., Ralph Bien, M.D., Roger Morrison, H.M.D., Lauren Deldin, Ph.D., Laura Carter, Spencer Bloch, M.D. Alan Schlacks, Ph.D., Brent Cox, M.D., James Stubblebein, M.D., Edward DeRosis, M.D. D. John Borchers, M.D., Barbara "Bobbi" Lambert, Ph.D., and Jacqueline R. Hampton.

For their support, encouragement and friendship, I owe much to my long-time friends Lee Beverly, John Mintz, Drew and Nani Prinz, Arv and Troyce Orbeck, and my brothers-in-law Jackie Chen and Michael Tseng. With great appreciation for their selfless work on my behalf, their unfaltering loyalty, and faith in my many projects, I want to especially thank my attorney, John Truxaw, my mother-in-law Nancy Lin, and my dear friend Ann C.W. Murphy.

I would also like to acknowledge my five doting sisters—Connie, Kay, Sydney, Naomi, and Gayle, who are living examples of strength and self-sacrifice; my brother Tommy, whose love of discovery and invention makes him depression-proof; my late mother, Naomi Mae, who devoted her life to her seven children, giving each a loving and secure childhood; and to my father, the Rev. T.F. Gardner, who kept his family together as a widower, and who helped me set the framework for an adventure into spirituality and healing, which will be the topic of a forthcoming book.

Finally, this book was the brainchild of my co-author, Art Bell, Ph.D., and I look forward to working with him on similar projects in the future.

━━◆━━

For Art Bell, Ph.D.:

Although I will owe a lifelong debt of gratitude to my professors at Harvard University and the University of Southern California and to my valued colleagues at Georgetown University and the University of San Francisco, my special thanks here goes to the more than 500 executives and managers for whom I have had the privilege of serving as a presentation coach and mentor. Their varied experiences with "speaker's nerves" and other presentation obstacles provided the genesis of this project, which of course has expanded far beyond the topic of performance anxiety. Each of these men and women know the progress they have made as business speakers, but they may not know how much they have given to me as a partner to their learning. It has been both a pleasure and a privilege to work with Dr. Gardner on this project. We hope that this book will be helpful both to those who suffer from anxiety, panic, and depression as well as to their friends, relatives, and work associates.

Contents

Introduction

Before we introduce ourselves, let us make a few guesses about you. First of all, you probably haven't selected this book for casual reading. The topics of anxiety, panic, and depression are rather important for you because you either know or suspect that you suffer from these conditions, or because a friend or relative suffers from them.

Secondly, you want the *whole* story on curing your problem (as best we can tell it within the scope of one book). You want to know how (or if) all the different therapies, advice from friends, counsel from your doctor, articles in newspapers and magazines, news items on radio and television, or spaghetti sauces (one brand adds St. John's wort to the recipe) really work. In one book, you want the tour of all the crucial information, along with many of the interesting nooks and crannies.

Finally, we assume that you expect this book to be true to its title—*Overcoming Anxiety, Panic, and Depression*. You're seeking paths for relief and recovery from these conditions that steal joy from life, that fill one's days and nights with anguish.

We plan to meet your expectations in these pages. In effect, we want to have a long, thoughtful conversation with you about the symptoms you or loved ones experience, about the underlying causes for those symptoms, and about the wide range of treatment that is now available.

In these pages, we hope to supplement or fill in the gaps with a conversation you may already be having with your doctor, mental health professional, spiritual counselor, or some other advisor. We will define terms you may have heard ("agoraphobia," "antidepressants," "obsessive-compulsive disorder," and so forth) and answer your questions about drugs, psychological counseling, herbs, vitamins, acupuncture, breathing, exercise, and meditation, among other topics.

This book **in no way** substitutes for the advice and care of a skilled medical or psychological professional. But the book can serve you well as a user's manual, explaining in plain language the workings of that amazingly complex world within your skin. We want you to understand anxiety, panic, and depression as well as you may now understand the rules of your favorite sport or hobby.

Information isn't all you will find in these pages. We also want to share sincere hope and optimism based on solid science. There has never been a time in human history when the age-old conditions of anxiety, panic, and depression were more treatable. The old, cynical "Rule of Thirds" ("one-third of patients will get better, one-third will stay the same, and one-third will get worse") no longer applies to sufferers from anxiety, panic, and depression who receive effective treatment. By understanding these conditions, grasping your options, and actively participating in your therapy, your prospects for improvement and recovery have never been better.

Trust is vital in any intimate conversation that goes to the root of *who* we are, *what* we fear, and *where* we can find help. We expect to earn your trust page by page. But, to begin to build that trust, let us introduce ourselves in our own voices.

———◆◆◆———

"Hello, I'm Dr. James Gardner. My 15 years of practicing general medicine have convinced me of the impact of anxiety, panic, and depressive disorders on the health of my patients. Of my present patient group of approximately 3,000, some 30 to 40 percent suffer to some extent from one of these disorders. I am profoundly humbled by the privilege of being intimately involved in their personal (and often painful) life experiences. Working in a large, solo practice in Marin County, California, I see patients of all ages, ethnic backgrounds, educational levels, and social status for a wide range of medical problems. Through my patients, I have learned the value of an open mind in considering ways of approaching any given illness. That openness to various treatment options is reflected in this book.

"On a personal note, I live with my wonderful wife, Patty, and our Yorkshire terrier, Gismo, on a quiet, wooded hilltop in Greenbrae, less than two miles from my clinic and the hospital where I was born in 1959. (You can visit us electronically at my Web site, www.docgardner.com.)"

"And hello from Art Bell. As a professor of management communication, I've worked during the past 20 years with hundreds of business and government leaders who suffer from 'speaker's nerves' and other related problems. These problems get in the way during presentations, meetings, and other performance occasions. (I am not a medical or psychological practitioner). Dr. Gardner and I have worked together on the situations faced by some of these men and women. That collaboration led to this book.

"If you would like to see my smiling face or just be in touch, please make contact through my Web site at www.usfca.edu/fac-staff/bell/home.html."

One other person speaks in these pages from time to time. Identified by the name "Barbara," she shares with you the personal and often painful details of what people go through when they are in the grip of anxiety, panic, and/or depression. We have included Barbara's eloquent diary of her own suffering as a way of putting a human face on what may seem to be a collection of medical terms and concepts. For many readers, Barbara's story here will release long-felt emotions of isolation, that someone else *has* experienced what I'm going through, and they made it out on the other side.

We won't invite you to sit back and relax for the journey ahead through these chapters. In fact, we expect the opposite. This will be gripping reading simply because these issues matter so much to you and so much to us.

Finally, we want to hear from you. Although we obviously can't offer individual advice or counseling by e-mail, we do want to know what you found helpful in this book and how we might improve the book for a future edition. Contact Dr. Gardner directly at www.docgardner.com and Professor Bell at bell@usfca.edu.

1 | Accepting Fear to Control It

For people suffering from anxiety, panic, and depression, it's hard to begin at the beginning in reading about these feelings. When "something hurts" emotionally, there's a natural desire to rush ahead to answers and solutions. Who has the time or patience for preliminaries?

There are no preliminaries in this book. The opening chapters are especially important in helping you understand the sources and causes of anxiety, panic, and depression. For many sufferers, such understanding becomes a major part of the answers and solutions they seek.

As an analogy, a sailor can rush ahead to stitching torn sails. But, for long-term solutions, even the most energetic stitching isn't worth as much as a moment's reflection on what's causing the sails to tear.

Therefore, we begin with first things first: how fear and stress lead to rips and tears in our emotional lives—and how such damage can be repaired and prevented.

Understanding the stress chain

Consider the chain of experiences that lead to anxiety, panic, and depression for millions of people worldwide. The first link in this chain of illness is *stress*. By nature, you probably attach negative connotations to that word: the stress of financial problems, the stress of work pressures, the stress of parenting (or being parented), the stress of dieting, the stress of broken relationships, and so on. Following this line of thinking and feeling, we should logically try to do away with stress entirely. It's bad, isn't it?

The question should be whether we would really choose a life *without* stress. For example, a new dating relationship, with all its stresses of risk, desire, jealousies, and insecurities, bristles with the energy and excitement of romance. A new career opportunity gets our juices going again after months or years in a sleepy job because new stresses are at play: the stress of working with new people, learning new skills, and making good impressions. We're stressed but invigorated. After all is done, usually we say to ourselves, "I should have done this years ago!"

You can add your own examples of stress seen in a positive light: perhaps the stressful allure of extreme sports (or *any* sports for some of us), the stress of a suspenseful movie or book (we *pay* to be stressed), or the stress of travel to reap the rewards of a memorable vacation. The list is endless.

In short, stress is the feeling that we're pushing against something — and building our strength, confidence, and character in the process. As we succeed at that pushing and manage to drive stress away temporarily, we feel a rush of pleasure. (In fact, pleasure has often been defined as relief from stress.) We work hard to drive away the stress of financial pressures and feel a sense of pleasure and accomplishment in seeing our piggy bank grow plumper. We push hard to exercise our bodies and feel a wave of pleasure (well, vanity) in standing before the mirror to see less of ourselves.

None of these common pleasures would be possible without the presence of stress. Like trees planted along a windy shoreline, we set down deep roots and grow into strong, resilient people because we haven't had it "easy" our whole lives. We feel that we have been tested by life events and have passed the test. We gain confidence that we meet life's challenges simply because we have met them successfully in the past.

Linking stress to fear

The next link in the chain of human experience also has a generally negative connotation: fear. Fear and its shadow, *worry*, are quite natural and common human responses to stress. You can think of fear as the alarm that goes off inside when you encounter stress. Worry, on the other hand, is waiting for the alarm to go off.

Here's an example: As a newly elected officer in a civic club, you're tickled pink by public recognition of your leadership abilities by other members of the community. But, when you learn that you have to give a 20-minute speech to more than 100 people at the next club meeting, you immediately feel stressed out. "Will I disappoint these people? Will I make a fool of myself? Will I appear nervous? Will I sound stupid?" These stresses are not at all silly. There is a risk, however slight, that all these things could happen. That risk produces stress.

In response to that stress, physical alarms begin to go off inside of you. As you look at the calendar and focus on the impending date of the speech, you feel your hands get cold and clammy. Your pulse, blood pressure, and breathing rate all rise. "My God," you admit to yourself, "I'm really *afraid* of giving this speech!"

At this point, fear is holding you back from fulfilling a responsibility and accomplishing something that you want to do. Before blaming fear for interfering with your plans, think for a moment about the function of fear in holding you back.

The alarms of fear, however uncomfortable, have the important purpose of saving our butts. All pilots learn the wisdom of the saying, "There are old pilots and there are bold pilots, but there are no old, bold pilots." We would have wished for a stronger emotion of fear within John F. Kennedy, Jr. before he took his small plane into inclement weather and then to eventual disaster.

Fear is the alarm clock that wakes us up to potential danger. Like any alarm clock, we wish we could shut the damn thing off and go back to sleep. But in the long run, we're grateful that it woke us up on time.

When fear turns ugly

Is fear our friend? Well, it is and it isn't. It certainly alerts us to possible threats. But our fear doesn't always have good timing and often has a lousy sense of proportion.

Let's talk about this timing of fear. For the sake of example, let's say you're staying at a rustic lodge near the south rim of the Grand Canyon. After breakfast, you plan to walk over to the edge of the canyon and peer down. Of course, you know that extreme fear will "go off" if you step too near to the edge of the canyon. You don't think about it, but you're grateful for this life-preserving emotion. However, what you didn't expect is for your fear response to begin clanging inside even as you take a few steps off the lodge porch. Your friends notice your hesitation. They ask you what's wrong. "I…I'm afraid to go any farther," you try to explain. Fear has stopped you dead in your tracks from seeing one of the wonders of the world.

In this case, the timing of fear was off. Just the *thought* of getting close to the edge of the canyon prompted fear's alarms many minutes before you were actually standing at the rocky brink of the Grand Canyon.

Now, imagine a life in which the timing of fear is almost always out of kilter. A life where you cannot do anything for the fear of what may happen.

Imagine common fears, such as those accompanying airplane travel, that go off days or weeks before a "can't-cancel" business trip. A man wakes up sweaty from nightmares and worries incessantly about the upcoming flight. When the day of the actual flight arrives, he has worked himself into an emotional storm, all because fear sounded much too early. And of course, those alarms sounded much too loud within.

Fear often has a poor sense of proportion. If you see a friend frantically thrash her arms and hands in response to her fear over a little bee, you might say, "It's just a little bee." Should we feel some fear over being stung by a bee? Of course. Should the presence of one bee buzzing idly around a soda can send us into the wild feelings of fear? Clearly, it shouldn't.

Dr. Susan Jeffers, in her famous book, *Feel the Fear and Do It Anyway*, puts the issue well, "What is stopping you, this very moment, from being the person you want to be and living your life the way you want to live it? The answer—beneath all the other answers—is fear."

What causes otherwise healthy fear to miss its timing so badly and leap so dramatically out of proportion? Some mental health professionals (including physicians, psychiatrists, psychologists, and a variety of counselors) view maladjustments in the fear response as a problem in the structure or biochemistry of the brain. Whether it has hereditary causes, environmental influences, or other factors, the brain isn't firing on all cylinders. From this point of view, the goal of therapy should be to discover the problem and then to use chemical, electrical, or physical means to repair the malfunctioning part of the brain. Proponents of this point of view are most likely to prescribe medicine to alter chemical functions in the brain, monitor its effectiveness, and make adjustments as necessary to alleviate suffering.

On the other side of the debate are equally distinguished mental health professionals, spiritual counselors, and others who view fear imbalances as the result of emotional blocks, psychological trauma, and related personality disorders. What needs fixing, they insist, is the way the person thinks, feels, and lives. Proponents of this position are most likely to address fear problems by talking to you and listening to you.

Linking fear to anxiety

Can you imagine your state of mind and jangled nerves if your noisiest alarm clock went off unexpectedly every few minutes? To say that your nerves would be "on edge" would be putting it too mildly. You would feel the uncomfortable sense of continual and undesired stimulation. You would yearn for a peaceful, rested feeling again. Instead, all you'd feel is a combination of exhaustion and the jitters. You'd have the vague sense almost all the time that "something's wrong" or "something's about to go wrong." Fear alarms—both loud and soft—would keep going off and your state of nervous arousal and sensitivity would become increasingly unpleasant.

Well, that's anxiety—a state of uncomfortable nervous arousal stimulated by fears that seemingly cannot be resolved.

The easiest anxiety to account for, though not always easiest to resolve, is "anxiety in the *now*." In this case, a person feels repeatedly and unnecessarily alarmed over some occurrence, object, or relationship present during the period of anxiety. A heart patient, for example, may feel profound anxiety during the first hours and days after a bypass operation. Each beat of the patient's heart felt—and certainly any skipped beats—can stimulate anxiety.

Perhaps more common, however, is the kind of anxiety that focuses on some future problem or threat, be it real or imagined. This is "anticipatory anxiety." In the painful days that often accompany divorce, either partner may feel quite anxious over undefined but deeply felt future threats: "How will my friends react? Can I make ends meet? Will the children adjust?" Athletes report similar anticipatory anxiety prior to a big sports event, often accompanied by sleep and digestion problems. (By the way, authors suffer with anticipatory anxiety when the stack of blank paper is higher than the stack of printed manuscript pages and the publisher's deadline looms. We heard through the grapevine that editors have similar anxieties.)

When anxiety has a focal point, we often describe the ongoing feeling of anxiety as "worrying." We somewhat obsessively play imaginary scenarios of threat and response over and over in our minds, teasing out details and implications with the result of increasing our anxiety.

In both of these forms of anxiety and related worrying, fearful feelings are directly attached to threats, however vaguely defined they may be. When the threat is removed—that is, when the big game is over or the bridge is crossed or the book goes to press—the anxiety subsides quickly. "What a relief!" we sigh. "It's over."

But some forms of anxiety aren't "over" so directly. "Unattached" or "free-floating" anxiety is more difficult to relieve because it focuses on no single threat or set of stimuli. Some people describe this form of anxiety as "feeling frazzled," "uptight," or "strung out." If you ask them why they feel anxious, their honest answer is "I don't know. It's nothing and it's everything." The severity of such free-floating anxiety can range from a general awareness that one is on edge to genuinely paralyzing anxiety states that keep people from working and, in some extreme cases, keep them housebound for fear of the outside world.

Linking fear and panic attacks

As described earlier, all fear sensations involve some physical component. The scientific basis for the lie detector, in fact, rests on the inevitable presence of some physical clues when the person being tested feels even slight fears about giving an untruthful answer. (Things such as perspiration, elevated pulse and breathing rate, changes in blood pressure, and so forth.)

Panic attacks are exaggerated versions of this physical response to fear. As if ready to fight some monster to the death, the body sends major organs into crisis mode. The heart and breathing rates soar, along with the blood pressure. If this sudden rush of physical energy were expended in wielding a battle ax against some fire-breathing dragon, we would probably be grateful for the powerful boost of adrenaline. But sufferers from panic attacks don't wield battle axes or slay dragons: They sit sweating in panic on a bench in the mall or in the restroom at their job. They feel intensely awful. After a panic attack, many sufferers recall thinking that death was imminent. (On page 21, Barbara describes in detail what her own panic attacks are like.)

In later chapters we will deal with the nature, causes, and treatment of panic attacks. It's enough for now to see panic attacks as one more link in the chain leading from basic fear. Just as anxiety may be attached to a specific threat or felt in a more free-floating way, so panic attacks can be provoked by specific events or circumstances, as well as by more general conditions.

One common venue for classic panic attacks is the airplane, particularly during take off and landing. Even though we are all statistically safer in an airplane than in our own homes (and certainly safer than in our cars), the rationality of the situation isn't the point for panic sufferers. They "know," at an intellectual level, they are relatively safe on the plane. But they also know, with equal or greater certainty, that sitting in a plane waiting for take off or landing stimulates truly horrible feelings of dread and physical suffering in them.

Not all panic attacks are so directly attached to defined situations. "I was walking my child to school," one female patient reports, "when I suddenly felt a huge wave of panic sweep over me. I had to sit down right there on the sidewalk and wait 10 minutes for it to pass. It scared me to death."

In this case, was the person consciously or subconsciously afraid of approaching her child's school, walking along the sidewalk, or holding her child's hand? Probably not. Some panic attacks appear to strike out of the blue, less in coordination with certain situations (such as the airplane) than with physical states (such as being overly tired or stimulated by caffeine or nicotine).

The final link: depression

"If you try to convince me there's *anything* good about depression," one patient told his psychologist on the telephone, "I'll come down to your office and give rose-colored glasses to you and everyone on your staff. This is hell."

Depression, like stress, fear, and panic, has a long and probably well-deserved rap sheet of crimes against humanity. From the Middle Ages on, this malady was known as "melancholia," from which stems our word "melancholy."

But "melancholy" hardly describes the experience of most depressed people. Depressed people aren't simply feeling sad, grief-stricken, or "blue." (In fact, we don't call depressed people "patients" because most depressed people do not [but should] seek medical or psychological help.) As later chapters will explain, the symptoms of depression vary widely. Most common, however, are profound feelings of despair, sluggishness, worthlessness, hopelessness, failure, physical torpor, and what one patient described as "mental nausea." In the words of George Brown, a psychiatrist at the University of London, "Depression is a response to a current loss, whereas anxiety is a response to a threat of future loss."

And what has been "lost" to cause such deep depression? People who are depressed often cannot articulate reasons for their suffering. If asked what depresses them, they frequently will respond with wordless tears or phrases such as "my whole life" or "just everything" or "I just don't know."

In many cases, the external circumstances of many depressed people is far from depressing. It is not uncommon for them to have wealth, social standing, supportive marriage partners and friends, and professional success. By contrast, many people living in poverty, facing abusive relationships, and struggling to find work don't fall into depression. (These generalizations are not intended to profile the typical depressed person, but instead to make the point that external circumstances alone do not cause depression.)

Some depressed people find themselves unwilling (and therefore unable) to get out of bed to face the day. Others feel utterly incapable of taking on and carrying through tasks that previously were easy for them. Still others plunge into prolonged periods of negativity and self-loathing, during which every silver cloud seems to have a black lining.

As dismal as this picture appears (and no doubt feels to depression sufferers), a growing number of voices in the mental health community are urging a reinterpretation of depression in at least some of its forms. In the same way that healthy fear alerts us to present or impending danger, depression may be the mind's and body's way of warning you of the brick wall at the end of a dead-end street of living. The mind and body seem to say in unison, "That's it. If you're going farther down that path, you're going alone."

Dr. Emmy Gut in *Productive and Unproductive Depression* suggests that the experience of "bottoming out" in depression, painful though it may be, is often a necessary staging platform for making important life changes. A drug addict, for example, who fails again and again to get clean and sober may need a bout of depression for recovery more than the well-meaning but disastrous "help" from an enabler. In this view, depression is not so much a baptism of fire as a baptism of fear. In the words of Joan Borysenko, author of *Fire in the Soul*, "...many dark nights of the soul are initiations into a new way of being. If the patient is willing to respond to the darkness, then an exciting, life-affirming newness can often emerge."

Dr. Gut has a conversion and recovery process in mind. If an addict needs to confront his substance abuse in the anguish of depression, why not the banker who has pushed himself throughout his life to please his parents and impress his friends and now in midlife finds himself with everything but happiness? Why not the woman who has assiduously "lived for her man" and threw away her own impulses for self-determination and freedom? Why not the teenager (an age group where depression is increasingly prevalent) who hates her gangly body, pimply face, and social awkwardness? Why not the senior citizen who has worked for a retirement spent dribbling a small white ball into a hole in the ground and now finds the game and his remaining years quite empty?

The question is not whether these people *deserve* depression. Which of us is to say who deserves rewards for life choices and who deserves punishment? Instead, the question goes like this: If you find yourself depressed, do you have to view that painful condition as proof of the continuing degeneration and degradation of your life? Or can you view it as a stop sign from the soul, with opportunities to turn in a different direction once you get going again?

The German Christian mystic, Meister Eckhart, expresses this viewpoint in his perception that "it is in darkness that one finds the light, so when we are in sorrow, then this light is nearest of all to us."

The idea of redemptive depression is easier to think and write about out of the presence of actual sufferers from depression. They often present themselves to their doctors and counselors as people on the verge of spiritual death, not spiritual rebirth. (We use the term "spiritual" here not with any specific theology in mind, but simply as a generally shared term referring to the "human spirit," including emotions, will, and perceptions.) Newer voices, such as those of Doctors Gut and Borysenko challenge therapists not to play unwittingly the role of enabler, allowing the addict to return to his drugs, the banker to his hated career, the woman serving every one of her husband's whims, the teenager to her Barbie fantasies, or the senior citizen to his aspirations of becoming Arnold Palmer.

Even if we grant that depression can present sufferers with an occasion for new life choices, the question remains whether the vast majority of these sufferers are capable of "conversions" in the ways they think about themselves and respond to life stresses. A century of research into behavioral conditioning insists that old dogs really don't learn new tricks very easily. In other words, people who have lived their way step by step into depression probably can't leap out of it, Superman-like, in a single bound.

That's where the various modes of therapy described in this book come to the rescue.

Summing up for now

Franklin D. Roosevelt's famous dictum, "The only thing we have to fear is fear itself," has been revised by mental health professionals: "Value fear for what it is telling you, then move on to live your life to the full."

Understanding the linked chain from stress to fear to anxiety, panic, and depression can help us make adjustments in our living, thinking, and feeling to quiet unwanted and unproductive alarms from ill-timed and misproportioned fears. Even our most painful personal moments in the grip of anxiety, panic, or depression can be viewed in a new light as a chance to rethink who we are, what we want for ourselves and others, and how we pursue our goals.

Barbara...

Anxiety, panic, and depression from the inside

From time to time throughout this book, I'm going to insert short vignettes of my personal experience with A.P.D. (my abbreviation for anxiety, panic, and depression). I am not a physician, psychologist, or psychiatrist.

But I am an expert, painfully so, on what anxiety, panic, and depression feel like. I've experienced A.P.D. as a daily part of my life since early teenage years. I have decades of personal experience in the trenches with anxiety, panic, and depression.

I don't tell these parts of my personal story to "bring you down." Instead, I offer personal details and memories in hopes that you will gain some comfort in finding a companion to your own struggles or those of someone close to you. Simply knowing that what you're going through isn't bizarre or particularly uncommon can be a relief in itself.

I remember as a young adult stumbling across a paperback written by a physician who treated agoraphobia patients (people who are afraid of open spaces). He included sad but moving descriptions written by the patients themselves of their complicated internal experiences of panic, anxiety, and depression. As I turned the pages I felt tears coming to my eyes and the word "Yes!" forming on my lips again and again. The experiences and feelings they were describing were very much like my own. These men and women had experienced the dark terrors and annoying life interruptions that I hadn't shared with anyone.

I wasn't alone! Simply knowing that other men and women had felt what I was feeling—and were receiving help—was an immense relief. The old spiritual song begins "Nobody knows the trouble I've seen..." I certainly felt that way at the beginning of my struggles with anxiety, panic, and depression. But others do know the trouble I've seen. In truth, a fairly significant wedge of humanity has struggled with the symptoms of A.P.D. in one form or another.

So my contributions throughout this book are a way of saying, "We're in this together. You're not alone." I needed that message desperately, and I share it with you by opening painful and personal details that may find echoes and resonating similarities in your experience.

For the record, I'm not a fictional character or an amalgam of Dr. Gardner's case files. Although Barbara is not my real name for obvious reasons of privacy, I am a real person living and working in the Bay Area of California. Each of the details narrated in these vignettes are from the truth of my experiences with A.P.D., as best as I can describe them.

2 | Do I Have Anxiety or Panic Disorder?

This chapter will get into the nitty-gritty of how labels (anxiety disorder, panic disorder, agoraphobia, obsessive-compulsive disorder, and many others) are attached to certain sets of specific symptoms. These pages will *not* attach any one of these labels to you, even if in your opinion the list of symptoms for a particular disorder seem to fit you like a child-proof prescription cap. Your physician or mental health professional reviews the big picture of your physical and emotional health before proceeding to specific diagnosis. Don't get there before your doctor!

If you suspect that you suffer from an anxiety or panic disorder from information presented here, discuss those feelings and symptoms with your doctor. If you have trouble talking about your symptoms or visiting your doctor for a sustained conversation, underline the portions of this chapter that seem to apply to you and take those pages along to show to your doctor.

You're not alone

An estimated 20 to 32 percent of patients in general medical practices suffer from clinically significant anxiety symptoms. Well, let's first define "anxiety," then specify what "clinically significant" means.

Anxiety is a subjective sense of unease, dread, or foreboding. It is "subjective" in that your doctor must rely on your self-report of how you're feeling. No mental thermometer can give a physician an objective reading of your anxiety level.

"Normal" anxiety involves accurate timing and proportion in response to stress. A stimulus, such as a near-miss accident on the freeway, a bumpy airplane flight, an important examination, or a public speaking occasion, produces common anxiety symptoms in almost all of us: cold sweat, rapid heartbeat, a flushed feeling across the face and neck, a lump in the throat, and general shakiness. Those symptoms disappear rather quickly, however, when the stimulus is removed.

This is not so with clinically significant anxiety symptoms, in which symptoms appear frequently and out of proportion to stimuli. In addition, these symptoms affect the usual patterns and habits of the individual's life (sometimes interrupting work, sexual function, normal sleep, recreational choices, and other aspects of living). Those who have clinically significant anxiety symptoms are given the diagnosis of Generalized Anxiety Disorder (GAD).

GAD is the most common of the anxiety disorders, occurring slightly more often in women and usually appearing first before age 20. Often a patient reports a history of vivid childhood fears and a predisposition toward shyness and social inhibition. The incidence of GAD is higher in those who have relatives with this disorder.

The most commonly reported symptoms of GAD are persistent symptoms of uncontrolled worry, restlessness, irritability, and apprehension. Patients often experience muscle tension and problems in concentrating. While patients with panic disorder complain primarily of autonomic symptoms (heart rate, shortness of breath, and cold sweats), GAD patients focus more commonly on symptoms such as insomnia (35 percent of the time), chest pain (33 percent), abdominal pain (31 percent), headache (28 percent), and fatigue (26 percent).

One of the most frustrating aspects of GAD syndrome for both patient and doctor is the tendency for anxieties to build upon one another and spawn new anxieties. For example, a person experiences anxiety symptoms and treats it by reducing his work schedule to three days a week. This change, however, leaves him not only with a new set of financial stresses but also with more free time in which to worry about his symptoms. The resulting new level of anxiety pushes him toward other maladaptive behavior such as excessive absenteeism from work, with additional anxieties, and so on.

The GAD patient is habitually pessimistic, worrying only that the worst will happen. GAD patients have a high frequency of substance abuse, primarily with alcohol, sedatives, and hypnotic drugs. Over 80 percent of GAD patients also suffer at some time in their lives from major depression and social phobia.

Physicians and other mental health professionals commonly apply the diagnostic criteria of the American Psychiatric Association in determining if a person has GAD. Those criteria require that the symptoms of persistent worry and anxiety have been present for more days than not during the past six months. The doctor must also determine that the symptoms do not stem from another anxiety condition (described below) and aren't the result of the physiological effects of a substance (a medication or street drug) or a medical condition, such as cardiac arrhythmia or overactive thyroid.

Panic disorder

Like anxiety symptoms, attacks of panic may or may not be associated with appropriate stimuli. Here's an example of an appropriate panic stimuli out of Dr. Gardner's garden of least-favorite personal moments. As a teenager, he had to have a wisdom tooth removed. His brothers and sisters lost no opportunity in describing to him how excruciating this procedure would be. Hyperventilating well in advance of being summoned to the dentist's chair, he felt nauseated, flushed, and clammy. When the dentist approached with what appeared to be a two-foot needle, your faithful author passed out cold.

By contrast, those with true panic disorder have attacks that are unpredictable and recurrent. In recent movies, Meg Ryan, Robert DeNiro, and Burt Reynolds have all performed credible enactments of panic attacks.

Figure 1:
Medical conditions suggested by anxiety symptoms

Cardiovascular
Acute MI
Angina pectoris
Arrhythmias
Congestive heart failure
Hypertension
Hypotension
Ischemic heart disease
Mitral valve prolapse
Pericarditis

Endocrinologic/metabolic
Carcinoid syndrome
Cushing's disease
Diabetes
Electrolyte imbalance
Hypercalcemia
Hyperkalemia
Hyperthyroidism
Hypoglycemia
Hyponatremia
Parathyroid disease
Pheochromocytoma
Porphyria

Gastrointestinal
Irritable bowel syndrome

Gynecologic
Menopause
Premenstrual dysphoric disorder

Hematologic/immunologic
Anaphylactic shock
Anemia
Chronic immune diseases

Neurologic
Brain tumor
Delirium
Encephalopathy
Epilepsy
Essential tremor
Familial tremor
Parkinson's disease
Seizure disorders
Transient ischemic attack
Vertigo

Respiratory
Asthma
Chronic obstructive pulmonary disease
Dyspnea (difficulty in breathing)
Emphysema
Pulmonary edema
Pulmonary embolus

Source: *Patient Care* magazine, August 15, 1999; p. 82

It is natural for both the sufferer and the doctor to seek situations that cause or contribute to these attacks. Let's say that a woman experiences a panic attack while driving her car. She may attempt to self-treat her condition by avoiding driving entirely, only to find to her frustration that panic attacks or the sensation that panic was imminent begin to occur in other locations and situations.

Left untreated, these recurring episodes of panic can close the woman's ordinary patterns of living one by one. She'll swear off driving. Then, after a panic attack in the grocery store, she'll let a friend do her shopping for her. An attack at church convinces her to stay home on Sundays. All too quickly, she finds herself housebound. In some severe cases of panic disorder, sufferers have retreated to their bedrooms after experiencing panic attacks in other rooms of the house. They become prisoners of their condition.

The American Psychiatric Association criteria for diagnosis of panic disorder are quite specific. Four or more of the following symptoms must be intensely and abruptly present and reach their peak within 10 minutes:

- ❑ Palpitations, pounding heart, or accelerated heart rate.
- ❑ Sweating.
- ❑ Trembling or shakiness.
- ❑ Sensations of shortness of breath or smothering.
- ❑ Feeling of choking.
- ❑ Chest pain or discomfort.
- ❑ Nausea or abdominal pain.
- ❑ Feeling dizzy, unsteady, lightheaded, or faint.
- ❑ Derealization (feelings of unreality) or depersonalization (being detached from oneself).
- ❑ Fear of losing control or going crazy.
- ❑ Fear of impending death.
- ❑ Paresthesias (numbness or tingling sensations).
- ❑ Chills or hot flashes.

The onset of panic disorder is usually during late adolescence to young adulthood, with the first attack commonly occurring outside the home. Onset in childhood and after age 45 is rare. Interestingly, the children of people with panic disorder have a four to seven times greater chance of developing the disorder.

Sufferers from play panic disorder often attempt to self-medicate, in many cases after repeated visits to health care centers and emergency rooms in an effort to find out what's wrong with them. Alcohol and benzodiazepines are often abused. More than half of panic disorder patients experience major depression at some time during their illness. They are prone to develop co-existing anxiety disorders, such as agoraphobia (30 percent of panic disorder patients), social phobia (10 to 20 percent), generalized anxiety disorder (25 percent), and specific phobia (10 to 20 percent).

This condition appears to spring from a combination of genetic predisposition, heightened sensitivity to nervous responses, and learned (that is, conditioned) patterns of behavior. Many panic disorder sufferers report that "fear of having another attack" is their primary source of anxiety and their reason for altering many aspects of their normal living.

Agoraphobia

This is a common manifestation of anxiety disorder, in which the person feels an irrational fear of being in places where he or she might feel trapped or unable to escape. A man, for example, might love to watch baseball on TV, but he'll never go to a live baseball game for fear of the surrounding crowd and close quarters for sitting. He has trouble explaining his feelings to his baseball buddies, who ask him again and again to accompany them to a game. Simply being trapped by all those bodies, especially when seated in the middle of a long crowded row, sends him into waves of anxiety symptoms.

For other people, agoraphobia makes attendance at concerts, church, or college lectures difficult or impossible. When they do manage to get themselves to these locations, they try to sit at the ends of rows or at the back of the room so they can slip out unnoticed if their anxiety symptoms build to the crunch point. Agoraphobics also usually hate being stuck in traffic, locked in a train or plane, or stuck in a tunnel or on a bridge.

Agoraphobics may become housebound as they avoid more and more places where anxiety and panic attacks have occurred in the past or are likely to occur. In one case chronicled in the *Guinness Book of World Records*, a woman allowed a benign ovarian tumor to grow to 303 pounds (the tumor alone) because her agoraphobia prevented her from leaving her home for treatment.

In Dr. Gardner's practice, a patient asked that he call on a family member who had not left his home in five years. "Out of shame during this time, he fabricated an elaborate web of excuses and feigned illnesses to explain to relatives why he could not leave home. If he stepped beyond the front door, he would become nauseated and vomit on the front lawn. If he pushed himself further and kept walking down the sidewalk, he would become disoriented and fall to the ground, unable to speak due to overwhelming dread. If someone came to his aid, he would not be able to answer simple questions such as 'What's your name?' or 'Where do you live?' He had not worked in six years since his panic attacks had started and paid a neighborhood boy to shop for groceries, passing them to him through a kitchen window. I spent an hour speaking with him and gave him a prescription for an antidepressant medication. Three weeks later, I was surprised to see him when I walked into my office exam room. He had driven himself for the first time in five years and was dressed appropriately for job interviews. Most gratifying was the familiar, relaxed smile of a patient who had succeeded after unspeakable struggles in taking back control of his life."

Specific phobias

These anxiety conditions involve persistent fears of objects or situations, exposure to which involves immediate anxiety reactions. These localized fears are called "specific phobias" and commonly include fear of needles, fear of heights, fear of insects and snakes, and fear of the IRS. (This is more than humor. The mere sign of the IRS postage mark [also known as the "bird of pestilence"] in some people's mailboxes can produce immediate and severe symptoms of anxiety.) For example, Dr. Bell has a good friend who is phobic about dogs. Whenever the friend comes to visit, Art's dog has to be shut away in another room. In fact, the friend's first question upon entering the house is always, "Where's the dog?"

People with specific phobia know that their fear is excessive and unreasonable for the stimulus at hand. A person with a phobic response to spiders, for example, would probably not be found trying to convince others that most spiders are dangerous. But that person will make every effort to avoid the dreaded stimulus to his or her fear.

There are several subcategories (or types) of specific phobias. These include animal type (fear of certain animals or insects, usually with onset in childhood), natural environment type (fear of storms, heights, water, and so forth, again with onset usually in childhood), blood-injection-injury type (fear of needles and other invasive procedures, with patients experiencing strong stimulation of the vagus nerve, causing cold sweats, slowed heart rate, drop in blood pressure, and sweating), and situational type (public transportation, bridges, tunnels, elevators, flying, and driving).

Specific phobias are often responsible for major life and career disturbances, as when an executive passes up a promotion for fear of additional air travel or when a businessperson in Marin County, California, refuses a better-paying job for fear of driving across the Golden Gate Bridge everyday.

Social phobias

Social phobias are distinguished by specific fears of social or performance situations, especially where the potential of loss of face, embarrassment, or causing worry to others is present. Social phobics resist leading meetings, taking oral examinations, making presentations, picking up new people at the airport or train station, going to cocktail parties, and attending social functions for civic or religious groups.

In his 1998 Broadway show, comedian Jerry Seinfeld cited a study that found that the number one fear of people surveyed was public speaking, with the fear of death coming in as the number two fear. "That means," Seinfeld observed, "given the choice, most people attending a funeral would prefer to be lying in the casket than up giving the eulogy!"

An estimated 10 million Americans suffer from social phobia (also known as social anxiety disorder). It is the most common anxiety disorder and the third most common psychiatric disorder after alcohol/substance abuse and depression.

Dr. David Sheehan, Professor of Psychiatry at the University of South Florida College of Medicine, emphasizes that social phobia "...is not shyness; people with this condition are profoundly disabled and significantly cost-burdened...People with condition have fewer social skills, than, let's say, you would find in panic disorder patients, who tend to cling to other people. So as a result, these anxious patients are more likely to get depressed. They're also less likely to marry people who don't have a social anxiety disorder. They're more likely to drop out of school early, be unemployed, and not seek work. They have difficulty interviewing for jobs, and they're likely to turn down promotions. They usually have fewer friends, and tend to cling to friends who might mistreat them....They are so anxious about meeting new people that they assume it's safer to stick with what they have regardless of whether the relationship is healthy or ideal. They tend to refrain from dating and are more likely to live with their parents as adults."

In certain cultures, including Japan and Korea, individuals with social phobia may develop an excessive fear of giving offense to others rather than of being embarrassed themselves. They may have extreme anxiety that eye-to-eye contact, blushing, or one's body odor will be offensive to others.

Typically, social phobia starts in the midteens. Onset may come slowly or may be abrupt after a stressful or humiliating experience. In adulthood, social phobia may come on quickly following a particularly traumatic performance situation, such as a public speaking experience that did not go well.

Stress disorder

Those who develop clinically significant anxiety symptoms after a traumatic experience are said to have "stress disorder." For example, a woman's encounter with a large, physically abusive man may cause her to feel generalized anxiety symptoms long after she is no longer in danger from the man.

If these anxiety reactions occur within a month after experiencing a traumatic event and resolve themselves within four weeks thereafter, the person is said to have "acute stress disorder." Traumas that stimulate this condition commonly include being the victim of rape or other violent crime, witnessing a horrific or tragic incident such as murder, having a near-fatal accident, or learning about the death or violent injury of a family member or close friend.

The person with acute stress disorder may have difficulty remembering the traumatic event or, alternately, re-experience it often in dreams, flashbacks, or recurring thoughts and images. Feelings of despair and hopelessness may lead to a major depressive disorder. If symptoms persist, acute stress disorder can develop into posttraumatic stress disorder (PTSD). If the anxiety reactions are delayed or recurrent, the person has posttraumatic stress disorder.

Many Vietnam veterans experienced this form of stress disorder. Traumatized by war events they observed and/or participated in, they tried to return to normal domestic life, only to find themselves beset by nightmares, sleep disorders, attacks of unexplained panic and anxiety, and other related symptoms. When these occurrences were separated from the war events by several years, many veterans had difficulty understanding the relation between the trauma of their war years and their posttraumatic stress disorder. Health care providers often had similar trouble accepting the case that emotionally troubled veterans were in fact victims of trauma years in the past.

Other events that may trigger posttraumatic stress disorder are violent personal assault, kidnapping, hostage situations, torture, surviving a disaster, being involved in a serious auto accident, and being diagnosed with a life-threatening illness. The criteria for diagnosing posttraumatic stress disorder are as follows: Symptoms must persist for more than four weeks and the disturbance they create must cause significant distress or impairment in occupational or social functioning.

Obsessive-compulsive disorder (OCD)

This disorder has received a great deal of press coverage, probably because its symptoms are highly visible and unusual. The person suffering from obsessive-compulsive disorder (OCD) uses ritualistic, repeated behaviors in an effort to chase away uncontrollable and obsessive thoughts and anxieties. Jack Nicholson in the movie, *As Good As It Gets*, portrays a character with OCD, as displayed in refusal to step on sidewalk cracks, obsession over tableware hygiene, and a compulsion to check locked doors. Other common OCD behaviors involve ritualistic washing or scrubbing of the hands dozens of times each day to avoid contamination, repeating a mantra or phrase over and over to relieve stress, needing to have things in a particular order,

Figure 2:
University of Miami Modified Maudsley Obsessive-Compulsive Inventory

You may wish to fill out this form and show it to your physician.
How much were you bothered by the following symptoms this week?

	Not at all	A little	Quite a bit	Extremely
I avoid using public telephones because of possible contamination.	☐	☐	☐	☐
I am more concerned than most about honesty.	☐	☐	☐	☐
I hate to throw old used things away.	☐	☐	☐	☐
I am often late because I can't get through everything on time.	☐	☐	☐	☐
I frequently have to check things (gas, electricity, water taps, doors, etc.) several times.	☐	☐	☐	☐
Daily, I am upset by unpleasant thoughts that come to my mind against my will.	☐	☐	☐	☐
I seem to worry more than others about health and safety.	☐	☐	☐	☐
My mind tells me to keep things (cans of food, boxes of detergents) even though they are empty.	☐	☐	☐	☐
I worry if I accidentally bump into somebody.	☐	☐	☐	☐
I tend to get behind in my work because I repeat things over and over again.	☐	☐	☐	☐
I use more than the average amount of soap.	☐	☐	☐	☐
It takes me longer than others to dress in the morning.	☐	☐	☐	☐
I am extremely concerned about cleanliness.	☐	☐	☐	☐
I find myself paying too much attention to detail.	☐	☐	☐	☐
My house is cluttered by old things I hate to throw away.	☐	☐	☐	☐
I am unduly concerned about germs and disease.	☐	☐	☐	☐
My hands feel dirty after touching money.	☐	☐	☐	☐
I usually have to count when doing a routine task.	☐	☐	☐	☐
Hanging and folding my clothes at night takes up a lot of my time.	☐	☐	☐	☐
Even when I do something very carefully, I often feel that it is not quite right.	☐	☐	☐	☐

Screening questionnaires can help identify people with obsessive-compulsive disorder. Although it is subjective and therefore limited, questionnaires such as the one shown here can help people realize the impact the condition is having on their lives.

Source: Dominguez RA, Jacobson AF, de la Gandara J, et al. Drug response assessed by the Modified Maudsley Obsessive-Compulsive Inventory. *Psychopharmacol Bull.* 1989;25:215-218.

having disturbing impulses such as shouting an obscenity in church, and checking and rechecking windows, stoves, and doors.

In most cases, individuals with OCD wish they could stop the recurring thoughts and images that lead to their behavior. When they attempt to quit their rituals, however, they commonly experience increased anxiety levels. Diagnosis criteria require that recurrent obsessions and compulsions are severe enough to cause significant stress or impairment and that they take up at least one hour per day. The onset of OCD is usually in adolescence or early adulthood and is at least in part inherited. Symptoms tend to wax and wane during the person's life, with the worst onset of symptoms occurring during times of stress.

Other anxiety-triggered conditions

Although space does not make it possible to give full discussion to the following conditions, we can at least define and show some of them:

Hypochondriasis is unwarranted fear of having a serious illness, despite appropriate medical evaluation and reassurance. Patients transfer their amorphous fears to a part of their bodies they can "blame" and then attempt to repair. Physicians often observe a pattern of migrating symptoms for hypochondriacs. For example, just when they are finally persuaded that they do not have a heart condition, they will then focus on potential kidney problems, and then on to suspected stomach ulcers, and then a train of other maladies. Unfortunately, it has become culturally accepted to mock hypochondriacs for the apparent absurdity of their search for an untreatable illness. In actuality, this irrational response to stress and anxiety is no more or less irrational than those to whom in our culture we accord sympathy, including people with panic attacks and/or periods of depression.

Trichotillomania is a disorder characterized by pulling out one's own hair, particularly in stressful situations. Although less common than hypochondria, this disorder has been around long enough to earn its own cliche: "Those kids made me pull my hair out."

Body dysmorphic disorder is a variant of obsessive-compulsive disorder, in which the patient has abnormal fears that body parts (typically nose, lips, chin, breasts, fingers, legs, feet, or sexual organs) are misshapen, ugly, or disfigured in some way by injury. Plastic surgeons often encounter patients with this disorder. Operations to "correct" the offending body part rarely succeed in satisfying the patient, whose anxieties and obsession stemmed from causes far different from particular body parts.

Anorexia nervosa is the fear of gaining weight, resulting in very unhealthy eating behaviors. The death of singer/songwriter Karen Carpenter from anorexia nervosa, as well as books, magazine articles, and movies on this subject have made the basic facts of this condition common knowledge. Patients with anorexia nervosa often attempt to control their intake of food by the practice of bulimia, that is, gorging themselves and then purging their meal through self-induced vomiting.

Separation anxiety disorder is an anxiety condition with its onset in childhood following actual or perceived separation from parents, siblings, or close friends.

Summing up for now

It's obvious that anxiety and panic disorders take many forms and that, in total, a significant portion of the population (probably more than 20 percent) fits the diagnosis criteria for one or more of the categories described in this chapter. Also apparent is the influence of family inheritance on many forms of anxiety and panic disorder and their typical onset of symptoms during adolescence or early adulthood.

These factors make us realize that "getting out" of panic and anxiety disorders usually isn't a matter of simply deciding to think and act differently (although courage and resolve do play a powerful role in recovery). Individuals with anxiety and panic disorders must usually be patient as they fight the good fight (with professional support) against maladies that have deep and pernicious roots in family history and in the individual's established life patterns.

For further information, take a look at the "Yale-Brown Obsessive-Compulsive Scale" **(Figure 3)**, which follows this chapter on page 37-39. If you are concerned that you are obsessive-compulsive, this rating scale may assist you and your therapist trace the roots of your problem. The "differential diagnosis of anxiety disorders" flow chart on pages 40-41 **(Figure 4)** can help you figure out where you stand if you feel that you may be suffering from anxiety or panic. (Of course, if you feel that you need to do this in the first place, you should contact a psychiatrist as soon as possible.)

Figure 3:
Yale-Brown Obsessive-Compulsive Scale

For each item, circle the number identifying the response that best characterizes your behaviors:

1. Time occupied by obsessive thoughts
How much of your time is occupied by obsessive thoughts?

When obsessions occur as brief, intermittent intrusions, it may be impossible to assess time occupied by them in terms of total hours. In such cases, estimate time by determining how frequently obsessions occur. Consider both the number of times the intrusions occur and how many hours of the day are affected. Ask how frequently the obsessive thoughts occur. Be sure to exclude ruminations and preoccupations that, unlike obsessions, are ego-syntonic and rational (but exaggerated).

Intrusion is:

0. Absent.
1. Mild (occurs <1 hours/day [h/d]) or occasional (occurs < = 8 times/d).
2. Moderate (occurs 1-3 h/d) or frequent (occurs >8 times/d, but most hours of the day are free of obsessions).
3. Severe (occurs 3-8 h/d) or very frequent (occurs >8 times/d and during most hours of the day).
4. Extreme (occurs >8 h/d) or near constant (too numerous to count and an hour rarely passes without several obsessions occurring).

2. Interference due to obsessive thoughts
How much do your obsessive thoughts interfere with your social or work (or role) functioning? Is there anything that you don't do because of them?

If patient is currently not working, determine how much performance would be affected if patient were employed.

0. None.
1. Mild; slight interference with social or occupational activities, but overall performance not impaired.
2. Moderate; definite interference with social or occupational performance, but still manageable.
3. Severe; causes substantial impairment in social or occupational performance.
4. Extreme; incapacitating.

3. Distress associated with obsessive thoughts
How much distress do your obsessive thoughts cause you?

In most cases, distress is equated with anxiety; however, patients may report that their obsessions are "disturbing" but deny "anxiety."

0. None.
1. Mild, infrequent, and not too disturbing.
2. Moderate, frequent, and disturbing but still manageable.
3. Severe, very frequent, and very disturbing.
4. Extreme, constant, and disabling distress.

4. Resistance against obsessions
How much of an effort do you make to resist the obsessive thoughts? How often do you try to disregard or turn your attention away from these thoughts as they enter your mind?

Only rate the effort made to resist, not success or failure in actually controlling the obsessions. How much the patient resists the obsessions may or may not correlate with ability to control them. Note that this item does not directly measure the severity of the intrusive thoughts; rather, it rates a manifestation of health, that is, the effort the patient makes to counteract the obsessions. Thus, the more the patient tries to resist, the less impaired is this aspect of functioning. If the obsessions are minimal, the patient may not feel the need to resist them. In such cases, a rating of "0" should be given.

0. Makes an effort to always resist, or symptoms so minimal doesn't need to actively resist.

Source: Adapted with permission from Goodman WK, Price LH, Rasmussen SA, et al. The Yale-Brown Obsessive-Compulsive Scale. *Arch. Gen. Psychiatry*, 1989;46:1006-1011. Copyright Wayne K Goodman, MD, University of Florida Brain Institute, 100 Newll Dr, Suite L4100, Gainesville, FL 32611

Figure 3:
Yale-Brown Obsessive-Compulsive Scale, continued

1. Tries to resist most of the time.
2. Makes some effort to resist.
3. Yields to all obsessions without attempting to control them, but does so with some reluctance.
4. Completely and willingly yields to all obsessions.

5. Degree of control over obsessive thoughts
How much control do you have over your obsessive thoughts? How successful are you in stopping or diverting your obsessive thinking?

In contrast to the preceding item on resistance, the ability of the patient to control obsessions is more closely related to the severity of the intrusive thoughts.

0. Complete control.
1. Much control; usually able to stop or divert obsessions with some effort and concentration.
2. Moderate control; sometimes able to stop or divert obsessions.
3. Little control; rarely successful in stopping obsessions; can divert attention only with difficulty.
4. No control; experienced as completely involuntary; rarely able to even momentarily divert thinking.

6. Time spent performing compulsive behaviors
How much time do you spend performing compulsive behaviors? When rituals involving activities of daily living are chiefly present, ask: How much longer than most does it take you to complete routine activities because of your rituals?

When compulsions occur as brief, intermittent behaviors, it may be impossible to assess time spent performing them in terms of total hours. In such cases, estimate time by determining how frequently they are performed. Consider both the number of times compulsions are performed and how many hours of the day are affected. Count separate occurrences of compulsive behaviors, not number of repetitions; for example, a patient who goes into the bathroom 20 different times a day to wash his or her hands five times very quickly is performing compulsions 20 times/d. Ask: How frequently do you perform compulsions? (In most cases compulsions are observable behaviors, such as hand washing, but there are instances in which compulsions are not observable, such as silent checking.)
Amount of time spent performing compulsive behaviors is:

0. None.
1. Mild (<l h/d) or occasional (< = 8 times/d).
2. Moderate (1-3 h/d) or frequent (>8 times/d, but most hours are free of compulsive behavior).
3. Severe (3-8 h/d) or very frequent (>8 times/d and compulsions performed during most hours of the day).
4. Extreme (>8 h/d) or near constant (too numerous to count and an hour rarely passes without several compulsions being performed).

7. Interference due to compulsive behaviors
How much do your compulsive behaviors interfere with your social or work (or role) functioning? Is there anything that you don't do because of the compulsions?

If currently not working determine how much performance would be affected if patient were employed.

0. None.
1. Mild; slight interference with social or occupational activities, but overall performance not impaired.
2. Moderate; definite interference with social or occupational performance, but still manageable.
3. Severe; causes substantial impairment in social or occupational performance.
4. Extreme; incapacitating.

8. Distress associated with compulsive behavior
How would you feel if prevented from performing your compulsion(s)? How anxious would you become?

Figure 3:
Yale-Brown Obsessive-Compulsive Scale, continued

Rate degree of distress patient would experience if performance of the compulsion were suddenly interrupted without reassurance offered. In most, but not all, cases, performing compulsions reduces anxiety. If, in the judgment of the interviewer, anxiety is actually reduced by preventing compulsions in the manner described above, then ask: How anxious do you get while performing compulsions until you are satisfied they are completed?

0. None.
1. Mild; only slightly anxious if compulsions prevented, or only slight anxiety during performance of compulsions.
2. Moderate; anxiety would mount but remains manageable if compulsions prevented, or anxiety increases but remains manageable during performance of compulsions.
3. Severe; prominent and very disturbing increase in anxiety if compulsions interrupted, or prominent and very disturbing increase in anxiety during performance of compulsions.
4. Extreme; incapacitating anxiety from any intervention aimed at morning activity, or incapacitating anxiety develops during performance of compulsions.

9. Resistance against compulsions
How much of an effort do you make to resist the compulsions?

Only rate the effort made to resist, not success or failure in actually controlling the compulsions. How much the patient resists the compulsions may or may not correlate with ability to control them. Note that this item does not directly measure the severity of the compulsions; rather it rates a manifestation of health—the effort the patient makes to counteract the compulsions. Thus, the more the patient tries to resist, the less impaired is this aspect of functioning. If the compulsions are minimal, the patient may not feel the need to register them. In such cases, a rating of "0" should be given.

0. Makes an effort to always resist, or symptoms so minimal doesn't need to actively resist.
1. Tries to resist most of the time.
2. Makes some effort to resist.
3. Yields to almost all compulsions without attempting to control them, but does so with some reluctance.
4. Completely and willingly yields to all compulsions.

10. Degree of control over compulsive behavior
How strong is the drive to perform the compulsive behaviors? How much control do you have over the compulsions?

In contrast to the preceding item on resistance, the ability of the patient to control the compulsions is more closely related to the severity of the compulsions.

0. Complete control.
1. Much control; experiences pressure to perform the behavior, but usually able to exercise voluntary control over it.
2. Moderate control; strong pressure to perform behavior; can control it only with difficulty.
3. Little control; very strong drive to perform behavior; must be carried to completion; can only delay with difficulty.
4. No control; drive to perform behavior experienced as completely involuntary and overpowering; rarely able to delay activity even momentarily.

The Yale-Brown Obsessive-Compulsive Scale is a reliable, objective, clinician-rated tool for determining the severity of both obsessions and compulsions. Scores on each item are totaled and interpreted as follows:
0-7, subclinical
8-15, mild
16-23, moderate
24-31, severe
32-40, extreme

Figure 4:
Differential diagnosis of anxiety disorders

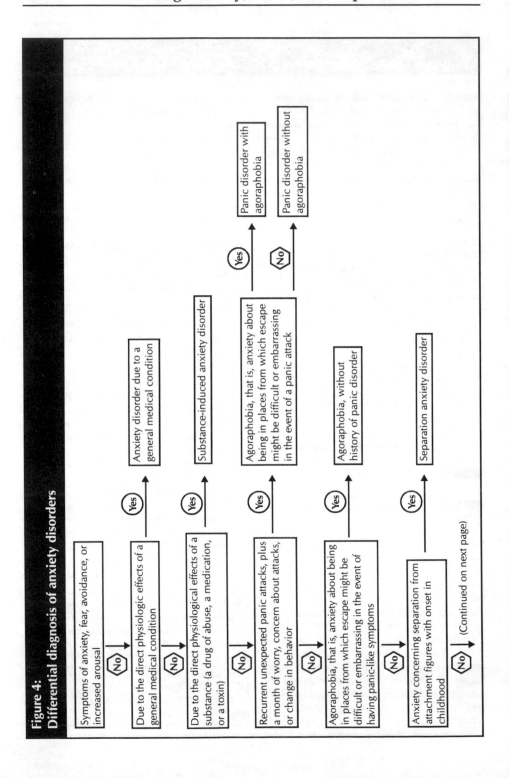

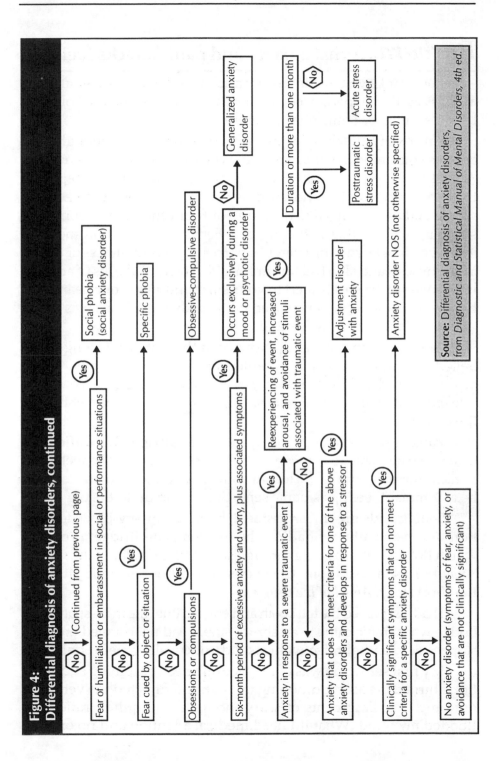

Figure 4:
Differential diagnosis of anxiety disorders, continued

Source: Differential diagnosis of anxiety disorders, from *Diagnostic and Statistical Manual of Mental Disorders, 4th ed.*

*Barbara...*What anxiety and panic attacks feel like

Let me take you inside anxiety attacks and related panic attacks, at least as I've experienced them. Your version—or that of your friend's—may be somewhat different.

An anxiety attack is not just a repeated worrisome thought that crosses your mind, such as a melody you can't get out of your head. Anxiety is experienced physically as much as mentally. To replicate the experience, call to mind a time when fright seemed to seize your whole body—perhaps like the surge of fright that may accompany stopping and rocking at the top of a Ferris wheel, or that moment when you first learned of a parent's or friend's serious illness or death. Your muscles and skin feel uncomfortable. Internal alarms of adrenaline make you intensely alert to your surroundings. Your heart feels hyperactive and oddly misplaced in the body ("my heart was in my throat"). Your breathing is rapid.

Got the feeling in mind? Now hold that intense feeling unrelieved for a few hours, and in duller form for day after day. That's anxiety disorder. You feel that you just can't get back down to a relaxed, rested state. It just doesn't go away, but instead ebbs and flows in intensity.

Panic is one notch up from generalized anxiety. It's difficult to describe true panic to someone who has never felt it. The feeling of panic is not the same as the feeling of fear, although fearfulness may be a dominant feeling as panic sensations ramp up to the big event.

Setting aside my embarrassment, here's a blow-by-blow description of a panic attack I had on the Golden Gate Bridge. (You can watch Robert DeNiro going through something similar in the movie, *Analyze This!* or read John Cheever's account of his panic attack in the short story, *Angel of the Bridge*.)

I had just passed the toll booth and entered onto the main span of the bridge when traffic came to an abrupt stop. I had not counted on being stopped dead on the bridge, with cars and trucks walling me in on all sides.

My first sensation was of my face and neck becoming suddenly hot. I turned the air conditioning up high and directed the vents full onto my face. Fragments of scary thoughts—all quite irrational—flooded my mind. What if I need medical attention and no one can get to me because of the traffic jam? What if I'm having a panic attack when traffic begins to move and I can't drive my car? What if I panic so badly that I have to get out of my car and abandon it while I lie prostrate on the bridge walkway alongside the traffic lanes?

These circumstantial thoughts were joined by quickly rising terror at what my body was doing. I felt my pulse racing wildly. My heart began throwing in extra beats. At this point, I felt horrible foreboding, truly the fear of seemingly impending death. Waves of adrenaline, like deeply uncomfortable thrills, caused electrical feelings across my scalp, neck and chest. I reached futilely and shakily to find a radio station—anything—to distract my attention from my experience. My fingers leaped back to my throat to feel my pulse, racing faster and faster.

I tried talking out loud to calm myself, saying reassuring things that doctors had said to me from time to time. Perhaps a minute passed in this full-out panic state. It was fortunate my car was stuck in traffic. I could not have driven in this state. I could hardly breathe. My kidneys ached from the force of blood pressure. Then the storm began to subside. Within a few minutes I was left pale, sweaty, and shaken, but able to steer the car on across the bridge once traffic began to move. I got to work completely exhausted and sequestered myself as best I could in my office.

This kind of panic event is deeply memorable (I'm tempted to say traumatic) and you find yourself willing to do anything to avoid repeating it. For many A.P.D. sufferers, this means avoiding certain places—the grocery store, gas station, or mall—where the panic attack took place. I had no choice but to cross the Golden Gate Bridge—it's the only route to my home. And, to be truthful, I don't feel I have conquered that bridge. I still have my good days when I breeze across the span without anxiety and other days when the painful and upsetting precursors to panic give me white knuckles on the steering wheel.

I had a well-intentioned psychiatrist at a large HMO tell me that "the experience of panic isn't really as dangerous as the things people do to avoid panic." I guess he had drug abuse in mind. In any case, I knew he had never had a panic attack. There is no form of pain—including childbirth—or other life distress I have ever experienced that I would not gladly take in place of a panic attack. Dangerous or not, panic attacks are pure hell to endure.

3 | Am I Depressed?

This chapter, like those on anxiety and panic, describes not only the general nature of the beast but also its specific stripes and species. You may not be interested in the medical terms for the various forms of depression discussed here. In that case, skim over the terms and focus on the descriptions of symptoms and other information offered for each category of depression.

On the other hand, you may be the kind of person who likes to call a radiator by its name instead of "that thing under the hood of my car." If so, we provide here a basic road map to the names doctors use to describe various forms of depression.

Above all, however, *don't be depressed* in reading this chapter. We are all fortunate to live in an age that marks a genuine renaissance in the understanding of and treatment for depression. Later chapters will describe and explain these forms of treatment. However, let's set the stage by first briefly surveying the landscape of depressive suffering.

Depression is one form of mood disorder. The word "depression" in popular use conveys the sense of despair, the "blahs," and the "blues." As we shall see in this chapter, some of the symptoms of depression don't fit that popular definition at all. Simply asking a person "Are you depressed?" may have little meaning if the term itself is not understood fully. Some extremely depressed people could truthfully answer, "Me, depressed? No way! I'm so full of energy I can't sleep and I can barely eat. If anything, I'm racing inside—not dragging." The first priority in this chapter, then, is to understand the full range of symptoms grouped under the umbrella term "depression."

Depression, like anxiety and panic, is serious business. Up to 15 percent of people with untreated depression will eventually succeed in taking their own lives. Most of these people will have seen a physician within one month of their death. Uncounted thousands more will die in accidents of one kind or another because they could not bring themselves to care about their own welfare or act in an emergency to save themselves.

When all forms of depression are considered, about three out of every 10 patients in general medical care fall into this broad category of diagnosis. For this reason, depression has been called the primary health problem of adult Americans—and one of the least-treated problems. This is especially unfortunate at a time when treatment for depression is safe, affordable, and available.

The symptom of anxiety is more common with depression than the symptom of a depressed mood. "Why are you prescribing an antidepressant drug for me? Can't you see I'm nervous and stressed out?" the patient may ask. In this case, the patient misunderstands the difference between a symptom and a syndrome. One can be depressed and have symptoms of anxiety, depressed mood, or both.

Depression: the sufferer's perspective

Before turning to formal definitions and descriptions of depressive disorders, let's hear directly from people who suffer from depression. What's it like to live inside the skin of a depressed person?

The answers to that question appear not only in Barbara's narrative on pages 57-58, as well as in the lists of symptoms posted by readers at the Web site, www.moodswing.org. Here are selected postings of symptoms as this book goes to press. All words, including those in parentheses, are those of depression sufferers:

- ❑ Reduced interest in activities.
- ❑ Indecisiveness (maybe).
- ❑ Feeling sad, unhappy, or blue.
- ❑ Irritability, dammit.
- ❑ Getting too much or too little sleep.
- ❑ Loss of, um, what were we talking about? Oh yeah, concentration.

- ❑ Increased or decreased appetite (my ex-mother-in-law's cooking notwithstanding).
- ❑ Loss of self-esteem, such as my understanding that I suck.
- ❑ Decreased sexual desire.
- ❑ Problems with, whaddya call it? Oh yeah, memory.
- ❑ Despair and hopelessness.
- ❑ Suicidal thoughts.
- ❑ Reduced pleasurable feelings.
- ❑ Guilt feelings, which are all my fault anyway.
- ❑ Crying uncontrollably and for no apparent reason.
- ❑ Feeling helpless, which I can't do anything about.
- ❑ Restlessness, especially when I can't hold still.
- ❑ Feeling disorganized (heck, look at my desk).
- ❑ Difficulty doing things.
- ❑ Lack of energy and feeling tired.
- ❑ Self-critical thoughts, which are natural when you suck.
- ❑ Moving and thinking sloooowwwly.
- ❑ Feeling in a stupor, that one's head is in a fog.
- ❑ Worries of financial ruin and poverty.
- ❑ Worrying about things that don't matter.
- ❑ Emotional and physical pain.
- ❑ Feeling dead or detached.

The humor included by sufferers in some of these symptom descriptions does not mean that depression is taken lightly. If anything, the humor here is what Freud called "tendency humor," in which a person conveys the real message veiled in humor. So when in the symptoms above a reader says "I suck" or "life sucks," those expressions probably reveal real feelings and personal judgments.

A major depressive episode

We'll begin by diving into the deep end of depression. A major depressive episode is obvious to all observers and to the sufferer. Interest in virtually all activities stops for a period of two weeks or more (one of the crucial diagnostic criteria for this category) and the sufferer experiences a markedly depressed mood. Symptoms commonly include loss of the ability to feel pleasure (anhedonia), withdrawal from usual activities, difficulty thinking and concentrating, anxiety, loss of energy, loss of sexual desire, feelings of worthlessness or guilt, sadness, speeding up or slowing down of usual body functions and movement, changes in appetite or weight (up or down), changes in sleep patterns (insomnia or hypersomnia), and thoughts of suicide. The person's social and work lives are significantly impaired.

During such an episode, if you ask the depressed person how he or she feels, the answer will probably be along these lines: "just very, very sad," "hopeless," "down in the dumps," "dead inside," "completely numb," and "no feelings at all." Their nonverbal aspects include downcast eyes, blank or pained expression, and a monotone voice. Sufferers commonly have slowed movements, weight gain, problems getting out of bed to face the world, and crying spells. Other sufferers, however, exhibit increased irritability, anxiousness, and even anger. In their restlessness, they may be unable to relax, eat, or sleep. They have agitated patterns of speaking and moving with repeated wringing of their hands.

Time of day often plays a part in how people experience depression. Symptoms are often worse in the morning, then taper off as the day wears on, sometimes intensifying later at night and interrupting sleep patterns.

Symptoms of the same sort: unipolar major depressive disorder

The term "unipolar" means "in one direction only." The sufferer experiences only the sad or numbing symptoms of depression, not those characterized by mood elevation, feelings of elation and euphoria, racing thoughts and little need for sleep (as described in the next page). This distinction is important in a doctor's diagnosis because it helps to define the appropriate treatment.

To be included in the category of unipolar major depressive disorder, a person will have experienced one or more major depressive episodes. Depending upon accompanying symptoms, the diagnosis can be refined to mild, moderate, or severe without psychotic features; severe with psychotic features; chronic; with postpartum onset (that is, after childbirth); with catatonic features; and with melancholic features.

Dysthymic disorder and "double depression"

Sufferers with dysthymic disorder have a depressed mood for most of the day (for more days than not), over a period of at least two years. During this period they do not have any major depressive episodes. However, they have two or more of the following symptoms: poor appetite or overeating, insomnia or hypersomnia (too much sleep), low energy or fatigue, low self-esteem, poor concentration, difficulty making decisions, and feelings of hopelessness. Many dysthymic disorder sufferers are self-critical, viewing themselves as ineffective or boring. If a major depressive episode occurs after a period of dysthymic disorder, the patient is often diagnosed as having "double depression."

Seasonal affective disorder (SAD)

Like anorexia nervosa, seasonal affective disorder (SAD) has become a star among the depressive disorders. It has been discussed with varying degrees of expertise in literally hundreds of magazine and newspaper articles, as well as television and radio shows. As a result, many people have self-diagnosed themselves with this disorder — often incorrectly.

Seasonal affective disorder is a dysfunction of circadian rhythms that typically occurs in the winter and seems to be caused by decreased exposure to full-spectrum light. Sufferers from SAD find that they crave carbohydrates, overeat, feel lethargic, and sleep much more than usual. SAD is much more common in women (60 to 90 percent). The disorder increases in prevalence as one moves farther from the equator. Symptoms typically subside in the spring and respond to increased light exposure.

Depression and periods: premenstrual dysphoric disorder

Brief mention should also be made of depressive feelings of varying degrees of severity that occur for many women in the late luteal phase of their menstrual cycle throughout the year (a few days to a week before the onset of menstruation). These feelings of inadequacy, physical unattractiveness, fatigue, deep sadness, and related emotions come on rather suddenly for many women with this form of depression, often "to the day" each month, in relation to their periods. For these women, the symptoms may disappear just as suddenly…until the next month.

Symptoms of extremely different sorts: bipolar depressive disorders

"Bipolar" means "two opposite directions." In discussing unipolar depressive disorders, we noted that the sufferer's symptoms all tend in one direction, that is, toward feelings of despair and inertia. In bipolar depressive disorders (formerly known as "manic-depressive disorder"), the sufferer experiences periodic and often dramatic mood swings from times of profound melancholy to other times of hyperexcitement, termed "mania."

Am I manic?

Viewed from the outside, a manic episode (one of the two directions for symptoms of bipolar depressive disorder) may look more like the cure than the disease. The person's mood is elevated — even elated or almost giddy. Far from hiding under the bedcovers, the person seems to be full of energy to the point of hyperactivity. Thoughts race and ideas stumble over each other in the rush to be expressed or acted on. The person feels little need for sleep. Grandiose and invulnerable feelings can send the person on uncharacteristic rampages, whether they be in the form of gambling sprees, sexual adventures, sudden career changes ("You can take this job and shove it!"), or breaks with family and friends.

These manic episodes typically occur in the spring or summer and are usually shorter in duration than their polar opposites, the "down" symptoms of depression. At their far edge, manic episodes can resemble schizophrenia with symptoms of gross delusions ("I'm Jesus Christ reborn"), paranoid thoughts, and auditory hallucinations (hearing voices). Symptoms of irritability and agitation are often present in manic episodes. In severe manic episodes, child or spousal abuse is often present.

More than 90 percent of people who have a single manic episode will go on to have future recurrences, most often right before or right after a major depressive episode. If untreated, the average sufferer will have four manic/major depressive episodes per decade of life, with episodes decreasing somewhat with age.

Mild manic episodes, or "hypomania," are borderline forms of mood swings that do not involve the more severe symptoms of mania (such as hallucinations and delusions). The change of mood in hypomania is observable by others close to the person, but sometimes is less apparent to the person himself or herself. To make a finding of hypomania as part of a larger diagnosis of bipolar depressive disorder, doctors will make sure the episode of mild mania lasts for at least four days and has three or more of the following symptoms:

1. Inflated self-esteem or delusions of grandeur.
2. Decreased need for sleep.
3. More talkative than usual or the feeling that one is under pressure to keep talking.
4. Flights of ideas or one's feeling that thoughts are racing.
5. Distractibility, in which attention is drawn off too easily to unimportant or irrelevant external stimuli.
6. Increase in goal-directed activity, including a feeling of urgency in achieving social, work, or school goals.
7. Excessive involvement in high-pleasure/high-risk activities (shopping sprees, sexual indiscretions, gambling, and so forth).

Happy highs and unhappy highs

Both mania and hypomania come in two flavors: euphoric and dysphoric. Euphoric sensations are characterized by feelings of being in love with oneself and the world, feeling boundless energy, talking a mile a minute, and spilling out grandiose plans and seemingly unattainable aspirations. This is the "happy high" that many popular magazines focus upon.

However, a less well-known but equally common kind of mania involves an emotional high with darker symptoms: agitation, anxiety, destructive tendencies or impulses, expressed or bottled up rage, and panic. This aspect of mania is termed "dysphoric."

The emotional tornado: mixed episode

The two poles of feelings described above for bipolar disorder can collide in a dramatic and often disastrous internal storm. In a mixed episode, the person experiences the symptoms of mania and major depression almost simultaneously or in rapid and alternating succession. Feelings of deep sadness turn to euphoria or irritability and hyperactivity, only to return within a short time to emotions of despair. During this internal storm, the person often complains of insomnia, appetite loss, and suicidal thoughts. Psychotic delusions may also be present. Needless to say, a mixed episode disturbance is often severe enough to require hospitalization.

When "it's not that bad": cyclothymic disorder

What if the symptoms are present for both manic and depressive disorders — but only in minimal degree? Mood changes fluctuate from despair to elation, but never involve a major depressive episode or a full-blown manic episode. The person seems temperamental, moody, unpredictable, or unreliable. Problems and misunderstandings are frequent in the person's work and social life.

If this fish-nor-fowl form of bipolar depression lasts at least two years, with symptom-free intervals of not more than two months or any manic, major, or mixed depressive episodes during the first two years, the condition meets the diagnostic requirements for cyclothymic disorder. It's not uncommon for this set of symptoms to overlap with those of borderline personality disorder. In that condition, the person experiences instability in personal relationships, generally

Figure 5:
Some conditions associated with manic or depressive syndromes

Neurologic disease
Parkinson's disease
Huntington's disease
Traumatic brain injury
Stroke
Dementias
Multiple sclerosis

Metabolic disease
Electrolyte disturbances
Renal failure
Vitamin deficiencies or excess
Acute intermittent porphyria
Wilson's disease
Environmental toxins
Heavy metals

GI disease
Irritable bowel syndrome
Chronic pancreatitis
Crohn's disease
Cirrhosis
Hepatic encephalopathy

Endocrine disorders
Hypothyroidism
Hyperthyroidism

Cushing's disease
Addison's disease
Diabetes mellitus
Parathyroid dysfunction

Cardiovascular disease
MI angina
Coronary artery bypass surgery
Cardiomyopathies

Pulmonary disease
Chronic obstructive pulmonary disease
Sleep apnea
Reactive airway disease

Malignancies and hematologic disease
Pancreatic carcinoma
Brain tumors
Paraneoplastic effect of lung cancers
Anemias

Autoimmune disease
Systemic lupus erythematosus
Fibromyalgia
Rheumatoid arthritis

Source: Dubovsky SL, Buzan R. Mood disorders. In: Hales, RE, Yudofsky SC, Talbott JA, eds. *The American Psychiatric Press Textbook of Psychiatry.* 3rd ed. Washington, DC: American Psychiatric Press; 1999:479-565

poor self-image, fears of separation and abandonment, and excessive anger when plans change.

Is it me or my medical condition?

The direct physiological effects of a general medical condition can be responsible for persistent disturbances in mood. Common medical conditions that may cause or underlie severe mood disorders include cancer, spinal cord injury, stomach ulcer disease, endocrine disease (diabetes, high or low thyroid, and adrenal gland malfunctions), autoimmune conditions (such as systemic lupus), painful or disabling rheumatoid diseases, acquired immunodeficiency disease (AIDS), other viral or infectious diseases (hepatitis, mononucleosis), end-stage kidney disease, degenerative neurologic diseases (Huntington's and Parkinson's diseases), cerebrovascular disease (stroke), and head injuries.

It is of the utmost importance that any patient with a mood disorder have a complete medical examination to rule out a medical condition. If such a condition is found, the patient should receive treatment not only for the condition but also for the resultant depression caused by the condition.

Is it me or my medication?

Many substances can be directly responsible for mood disorders. Some standard medications, including diet pills, stimulants, steroids, and antidepressants, can induce manic-like mood disturbance, as can other treatments for depression such as EDS (electroencephalogram-driven stimulation) or ECT (electroconvulsive therapy). Other medications including birth control pills, sedatives, and anxiety medications can cause a depressed mood.

Environmental substances, such as heavy metals, toxins, gasoline, paint, insecticides, nerve gases, carbon monoxide, and carbon dioxide can cause a wide range of mood and perception disturbances. Doctors recognize substance-induced mood disorder by the direct relation between the presence of the substance and the related symptoms. When the offending substance is removed, the symptoms disappear.

🐚 Summing up for now

Depression in all its manifestations is a serious disturbance to joyful, healthy living. In its advanced form, the illness can be life threatening. Because symptoms of depression overlap with symptoms of many other conditions and diseases, people who suspect they suffer from depression should seek a thorough medical examination as a first step in tackling the problem.

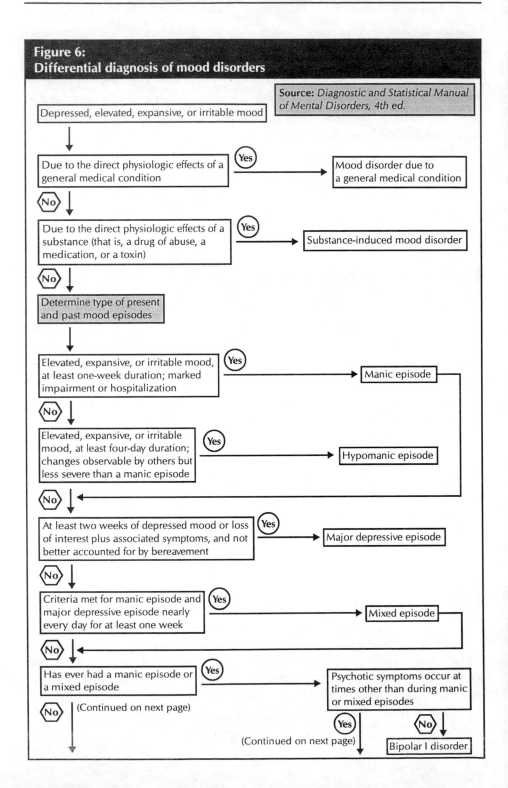

Figure 6:
Differential diagnosis of mood disorders

Source: *Diagnostic and Statistical Manual of Mental Disorders, 4th ed.*

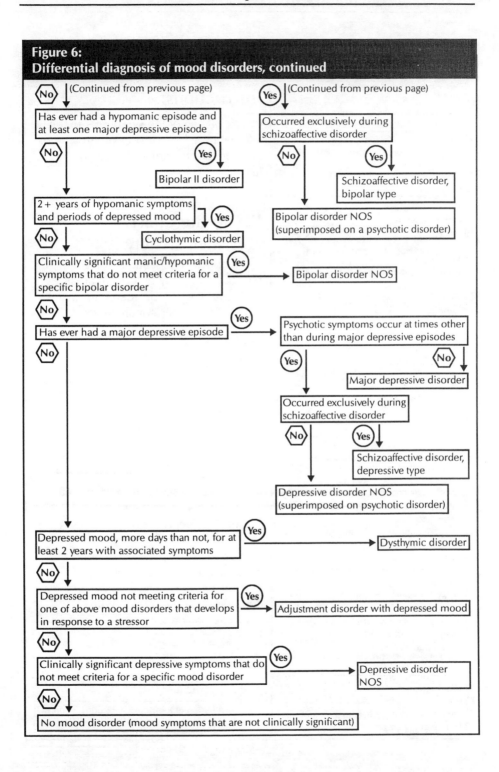

Figure 6:
Differential diagnosis of mood disorders, continued

Figure 7:
The Focus Well-Being Chart

☐ Fever
☐ Repetitive, senseless thoughts
☐ Repetitive, senseless behaviors
☐ Fainting or feeling faint
☐ Tremors, trembling, or shakiness
☐ Seizures
☐ Easy bruising
☐ Skin rash

(1)
☐ Violent behavior
☐ Constant worry
☐ Irritability
☐ Tension
☐ Headache
☐ Feeling in a dreamlike state
☐ Fearful feelings
☐ Fear of losing control
☐ Jumpiness
☐ Restlessness
☐ Sweating
☐ Dizziness/light-headedness
☐ Keyed up/on edge

(2)
☐ Agitation
☐ Nervousness
☐ Trouble concentrating
☐ Insomnia/trouble sleeping
☐ Decrease in sex drive
☐ Trouble making decisions

(3)
☐ Sad/depressed
☐ Lack of/loss of interest in things
☐ Helpless feelings
☐ Fatigue—lack of energy
☐ Weakness
☐ Increase or decrease in appetite
☐ Increase or decrease in weight
☐ Frequent crying or weeping
☐ Frequent thoughts of death or suicide
☐ Worthless feelings
☐ Excessive feelings of guilt
☐ Hopeless feelings
☐ Feeling life is not worth living
☐ Sleeping too much
☐ Frequent negative thinking

☐ Memory problems
☐ Fear of doing something uncontrollable
☐ Fear of dying
☐ Chills
☐ Seeing or hearing things that are not real
☐ Fear of going crazy

Instructions:

Check off any of the symptoms to the left that have been most bothersome or have occurred frequently during the last four weeks.

Key to the Chart:
Persistent anxiety

If you checked "Constant worry," plus three other symptoms in areas 1 or 2, you may be considered for a diagnosis of persistent anxiety.

Depression with associated anxiety

If you checked any symptoms in area 2, plus either of the first two symptoms in area 3, you may be considered for a diagnosis of depression with associated anxiety.

Depression

If you checked six symptoms in area 3, you may be considered for a diagnosis of depression.

Of course, a complete evaluation is necessary to firmly establish a diagnosis of persistent anxiety, depression, or depression with associated anxiety.

Source: Reprinted with permission of Bristol-Myers Squibb Neurosicence

Barbara... Anxiety, panic, depression, and guilt

I feel terribly guilty about allowing myself to remain in the grip of anxiety, panic, and depression.

If I had a broken arm, I wouldn't feel deeply guilty and apologetic. I might view my temporarily disabled limb as an inconvenience or, perhaps, as a silly mistake from skiing above my skill level. But I certainly wouldn't agonize over it as my personal failing and flaw. If anything, I'd get people to sign my cast and make a joke of it.

That's not so with A.P.D. I feel awful that I can't rely on myself to do the things others do with such pleasure. Why can't I go with my husband to the company picnic and expect not only to feel good but to have a good time? I'll be wondering when waves of nervous feeling are going to verge over into a full-blown panic attack. I'll be feeling my pulse to see if I'm racing inside, and then worry about that. I'll be forcing a smile for people I meet and trying to appear "normal."

I feel that I've dropped the ball by not grabbing hold of this affliction and wrestling it to the ground, as I have with other challenges in my life. Why do I let "it" creep on and on in my life, corrupting every wedding and dinner party I've attended in recent years (or sent my regrets for at the last minute)?

When I do have panic attacks or times when "nerves" make it impossible for me to continue (whether in a business function, a recreational pursuit, or whatever), why do I find myself apologizing to everyone and anything in sight? ("I'm so sorry. I'm really okay. No, don't call an ambulance. I'm so, so sorry to interrupt things. Yes, I'll be okay in a few minutes. This is so ridiculous. I'm *so* sorry!")

I would never say such things about a broken arm, a sudden attack of asthma, or a fainting spell. In those cases, I—along with everyone around me—would recognize that I have something wrong with me. I would make whatever adjustments I needed to and change life to fit my disability. If I had a broken arm, I wouldn't try to pitch at a baseball game. If I had asthma, I wouldn't climb Mount Everest.

But that's exactly what I seem to be doing with my A.P.D. disability. I'm putting myself in circumstances where I'm doomed to experience painful fears and waves of physical panic over and over again. Instead of learning from the pain, I go on and on trying to "fake" a normal life.

Fly to the Caribbean? Sounds great, Jim! (I'm scared stiff.) Take a hike together through a national forest? Wonderful, kids! (Each step will take me further from hospital emergency rooms or at least a bed where I can lie down and collect myself. If I have an "attack" miles from nowhere, how will I get back? What will I do when I'm sitting there under a tree, exhausted from panic with my family and friends staring at me, wondering what is the matter. I hate to cause them worry, and I feel extremely guilty when I do.

Somehow I've come to believe that my experiences of A.P.D. are my fault—that I could change everything back to "normal" if only I had more courage and will power, or if I had exerted more effort in finding the right therapist or magic pill to make all this go away. I consider my feelings to be my failure, and I feel terribly guilty for the havoc those feelings have caused for me and for others in my life.

4 | Why Am I This Way?

Our priorities are interesting when we experience pain, be it mental or physical. We turn first to seek relief. But even in the process of seeking relief we, (as *homo sapiens* — "wise" creatures), also seek knowledge about our pain. What causes it? Something inside us? Something outside us? Both?

People struggling with anxiety, panic, and depression want relief from the emotional pain and the physical symptoms that accompany it. But they also ask themselves (and their doctors) searching questions: "Am I to blame? Am I doing all this to myself? Do I simply have bad genes, a weak character, or a lousy childhood? What causes my emotional distress? Is it my job stress? My spouse?"

Looking back for answers

The bad news is that we don't yet know in any final way what factors or combination of factors causes anxiety, panic, and depression. However, the good news is that we're getting much closer to those answers and explanations.

To put our new knowledge about anxiety, panic, and depression in perspective, it's worthwhile to look back over our shoulder for a moment to see how other men and women in former eras struggled valiantly to find causes and solutions for these emotional disturbances. Even a brief glance at the past can persuade us that the problem is not new. Millions of our ancestors felt the same mysterious grip of anxiety, panic, and depression—and left us valuable lessons from their experience. This past can make us feel fortunate, even in the midst of our suffering, to be alive at a time when these maladies are more treatable than ever before. The past is a veritable Madame Tussaud gallery of horrors and heroes. What doesn't work in healing emotional distress is preserved for all to see and avoid. At the same time, brilliant minds also shine out like beacons across the ages to enlighten our own search for answers.

Heaven, hell, and the humors

In ancient Greece, mental disorders were thought to be the result of divine punishment. If you were depressed in that era, you could blame yourself if you knew you had offended the gods in some way. Or, if innocent, you could blame the fickleness of the gods. In either case, you were the victim of divine action.

Against that cultural and theological backdrop, it took considerable courage in the fifth century B.C. for Hippocrates (father of modern medicine and author of the Hippocratic Oath taken by physicians to this day) to call temple priests "swindlers, charlatans, and magicians" who took advantage of the emotionally weak and vulnerable. Hippocrates' own father was one of these priests who attempted to heal by religious ritual. Probably to his father's great dismay, Hippocrates proposed that both mania and melancholia (depression) were disorders of the brain—not punitive whims of the gods.

Specifically, he blamed the imbalance of natural body fluids for emotional disturbance. The brain, he said, is influenced by the presence of four humors: blood, phlegm, black bile, and yellow bile. When these fluids were in the wrong place or wrong proportion, illness (both physical and emotional) was the result. An excess of yellow bile could overheat the brain to the point of mania and rage. Black bile, on the other hand, tended to chill the brain and cause melancholic feelings.

With considerable insight, Hippocrates observed that external stresses could impact the apparent internal proportions and workings of the humors. For the first time, emotional disturbances were seen as complex phenomena involving both internal and external factors.

Panic and hysteria in Hippocrates' time were regarded as feminine disorders (whence our word "hysterical," from the Greek word for uterus). The uterus was thought to be corrupted if deprived of sexual activity. The uterus would then travel throughout the body, causing a variety of ailments. For all the anatomical nonsense of this theory, it expressed 2,000 years before Freud the notion that sexual impulses and experiences were somehow connected with emotional struggles.

Through the Roman physician Galen (second century A.D.) the humoral theory of health and emotion came down through the Middle Ages to the Renaissance and Robert Burton's vastly influential work, *The Anatomy of Melancholy* (1641). Burton catalogued all the popular theories of his day regarding the causes of depression. Many people (and most priests) still saw the illness as proof of divine displeasure or the work of devils. (The Roman Catholic ritual of exorcism remains to this day a testimony to the long-lived idea that "the devil made me do it.") Others explained depression as the result of one or more of the following: substance abuses (in the day, excessive wine, garlic, onions, and spices), too much heat from the sun, too much mental effort in studying, too much loneliness and idleness, or head injuries of various kinds. Treatment consisted largely of attempting to purge or readjust the balance of humors by induced vomiting, diarrhea, bloodletting, and the use of alcohol and opium (often in combination).

With the discovery of the circulation of blood by Pinel and Harvey in the 18th century came a new interest in the brain and nervous system. What could be carried to the brain by blood and neural channels to cause emotional imbalance? "Nerve juices" were postulated, and treatment shifted toward keeping those juices as pure and vital as possible. Spa water was recommended to strengthen the nerves and medications to relieve sleep disorders became commonplace.

The notion of "nerve juices," of course, was not far removed from the older idea of humorous fluids. Could there be another explanation? A true revolution in the interpretation of emotional ills was championed by Pinel in the 19th century. He argued for what he called the "moral" causes of depression and anxiety, among which he included frustrated ambition, unrequited love, and domestic problems. The cure for these unhappy experiences, he felt, did not lay in bloodletting or vomiting, but in surrounding the patient with pleasant diversions and entertainment.

Contributing to Pinel's theories of environmental influence was the late-19th-century theory of neurasthenia, or "exhaustion of the nervous system." Just as Pinel felt that a person's emotions could be exhausted by painful life experiences, so a number of prominent Victorian physicians proposed that the nerves themselves, much like overused biceps, could experience periods of weakness and exhaustion. Tonics, potions, and mild electric stimulation became the order of the day for strengthening the nerves in an effort to banish anxiety, panic, and depression.

Although hardly a household name then or now, a brilliant German psychiatrist, Emil Kraepelin, laid much of the groundwork before the turn of the century for modern psychiatry and psychology. He insisted on studying mental disorders by observing behaviors and symptoms, then classifying them systematically. For example, his classification scheme had separate categories for mental disorders due to medical conditions and those due to substance abuse. He made the connection between mania and melancholy, calling it "manic-depressive psychosis." He defined what he called "war neurosis," now called posttraumatic stress disorder.

Born the same year as Emil Kraepelin, Sigmund Freud drifted away from neurological explanations for anxiety, panic, and depression to a new model based on stages of human development. Mental imbalances and illnesses, Freud felt, were the inevitable result of early childhood conflicts stemming from parental suppression through disapproval and punishment of the child's natural aggressiveness and sexual drives. When stress occurs in adult life, Freud theorized, the person tries to deal with resulting anxiety by regressing to childhood emotions and behaviors. Obsessive-compulsive disorder, for example, is interpreted as an anxiety-ridden effort to "do it right" and harkens back to the anal stage of toilet training, with its challenges to self-control and traumatic memories of parental stresses.

In opposition to Freud, two generations of cognitive behavioral doctors and researchers have followed the insights of B.F. Skinner and others in arguing that much mental disturbance is learned behavior. As such, it can be gradually "unlearned" and replaced by new, more healthful patterns of thinking and feeling. Put simply, if Pavlov's dogs can learn to salivate at the sound of bell, why can't human beings be conditioned (both positively and negatively) to respond emotionally to internal and external stimuli? Much of the self-help literature crowding the psychology or mental health shelves in the bookstore are based on this learning model of mental health.

The general idea is as follows: Think differently about your problem and it will disappear (or at least lessen) in intensity. Since all reality is assumed to be personally constructed, these books propose to help readers remodel that construction for greater happiness and less emotional pain.

Right to the present: what we have learned

Although it is difficult to summarize in a few pages the stunning work of thousands of modern researchers, doctors, philosophers, and theologians, we can at least dip into the mainstreams of their thinking by reviewing how genetic influences, temperament predispositions, parental/childhood experiences, and stress (external and internal) all play roles in the cause of anxiety, panic, and depression.

Genetic influences

It has long been known that anxiety, panic, and depression run in families. With recent advances in molecular genetics, investigations are presently underway to map genes that influence these disorders from generation to generation. At present, our most reliable information comes from close studies of family members and particularly from twin studies. (The logic goes like this: If twins are separated soon after birth and still develop similar emotional disorders, there's good evidence that the cause of those disorders is genetic rather than environmental.)

One famous study of families by R.B. Goldstein and colleagues in 1997 showed the powerful influence of genetic inheritance in early-onset panic disorder. The sons and daughters of parents who developed panic disorder before age 20 were more than three times more likely to develop panic disorder themselves than were children of parents who had later onset of panic disorder.

Similarly, "first-degree relatives" (brothers, sisters, parents, children) of a person with major depressive disorder are up to three times more likely to get the disorder themselves. First-degree relatives of those with bipolar disorder have up to 25 percent higher risk of developing either bipolar or major depressive disorder than people in the general population.

A family inheritance pattern has also been established with social phobia and, amazingly, with specific phobia. A first-degree relative of a person who fears animals, for example, is more likely to also develop a specific phobia for animals, although not necessarily the same animal. Fear of needles, blood, and injury have particularly strong patterns of inheritance.

In all such studies, researchers try to establish the "degree of concordance" between related people. Concordance simply means that both subjects in a study have a particular trait or disorder. In studying twins, for example, a disorder would be found to be completely genetic if both identical twins had it (since identical twins have identical genes). The concordance between these twins would be 100 percent. If the same disorder were found in fraternal twins, where only 50 percent of genetic material is shared, the concordance would be 50 percent.

This background information is necessary to appreciate the degree to which genetics play a powerful role in anxiety, panic, and depression. In a study by Torgersen in 1983, identical twins were found to have a 60 percent concordance rate for panic disorder but only a 17 percent concordance rate for generalized anxiety disorder (GAD). Carey and Gotesman's 1981 study showed a 33 percent concordance rate for obsessive-compulsive disorder in identical twins, and a later study (Rasmussen and Zahn, 1984) showed a 57 percent concordance rate for this disorder.

But couldn't twins develop similar disorders not because of genetics but because they were raised under the influence of similar stresses and other environmental factors? For this very reason, studies of identical twins separated at birth are crucial for our understanding of inherited tendencies toward emotional illness. In the Minnesota Separated Twin Study of 1982, nine pairs of identical twins reared apart were found in which at least one of each pair had a specific phobia. In six of the nine cases (67 percent), the other twin also had a phobia. In some cases, it was the same kind of phobia.

Twin studies by Dr. Kendler and his colleagues in the early 1990s used large samples of twins with anxiety and depressive disorders. In analyzing the data, Kendler's team came to the conclusion that generalized anxiety disorder and major depressive disorder shared a common genetic factor — you could "get it" from parents and other ancestors. But the study found that whether you developed anxiety disorder or depressive disorder was determined by your temperament and environmental factors as you matured. In short, you were predisposed to get "it" by genetic inheritance, but what "it" was depended more on you and your life than on your parents.

What are we to feel about the loading of the genetic dice against us in inherited tendencies toward anxiety, panic, and depression? "I'm doomed," a patient recently complained. "Both my mother and my father had major depressive episodes at some time in their lives." Are you doomed? Hardly — but you should feel alerted. No genetic background available makes it certain that we will develop the emotional ills suffered by our parents. Genetic information is best used to remind ourselves that we are more at risk for anxiety, panic, and depression than others in the general population, and that we should act early to seek professional help if we observe tell tale symptoms of these illnesses.

We should also take time to learn about the emotional health of our parents and first-degree relatives. Often, adult children do not really know much about mom or dad's emotional health history until they become directly responsible for the management of their parents' health care in old age. While their children are growing up through their young to their adult years, parents may assiduously hide any information about emotional distress, episodes of depression, or bouts with anxiety and panic. "Why worry the children," the logic goes. "They have their own lives and concerns." It is not uncommon for a first-time patient to not answer the family history questions correctly regarding anxiety, panic, and depression to a physician or mental health professional. The patient does this, only to discover that, hidden from view, the mother had experienced panic attacks since young adulthood and the father had been hospitalized twice with depression. Tragically, emotional ills are still treated by some people as a scarlet letter "A"; something to be ashamed of and to hide from—especially from those one loves most. If their children knew the family predisposition toward a particular emotional ailment, they could act sooner and more wisely to protect themselves against the disorder.

Temperament

Temperament is our disposition present at birth. Every mother has a feeling from the start whether her infant will be calm and placid or crabby and difficult. At the forefront of temperament research is Jerome Kagan of Harvard University. He describes four basic types of personalities: timid, bold, upbeat, and melancholic. He relates each to a different pattern of brain activity.

About 15 to 20 percent of children, says Kagan, are born timid. They have a more responsive neural circuitry that is easily aroused by even mild stress. Compared to other children, their hearts beat faster when confronted by new or strange situations. As infants, they are more finicky about new foods, act shy around strangers, and are reluctant to explore anything unfamiliar. As children, they shrink away from social situations, participate less in class activities, and find themselves less popular than other children. Throughout life, they view new people and situations as potential threats. As adults, they are prone to being uncomfortable where they may be subject to critical scrutiny and the judgment of others (for example, giving a speech or performing in public).

The neurochemistry of timidity seems to center in a part of the brain known as the amygdala. This area is more easily aroused in those prone to fearfulness, and arousal of the amygdala causes feelings of anxiety and unease. The more easily this brain area is aroused, the more the person will shy away from anything that triggers its activation.

Kagan found that about 40 percent of the general population were born with a bold temperament. Bold individuals have a high threshold for triggering the amygdala. Therefore, they are less easily frightened, more outgoing, and more eager to interact socially. This temperament is advantageous in building up the growing child's self-esteem. Things go well with friends and reinforce the child's self-image as a likeable, worthwhile individual.

Those born with the cheerful, upbeat temperament are naturally easygoing and optimistic. They are hard to rile and fun to be with. They enjoy life and share their joy naturally and often with others. Richard Davidson, psychologist at the University of Wisconsin, discovered that those with a higher level of activity in the left frontal lobe of the brain, compared to the right, are cheerful by temperament. They rebound easily from setbacks and find interest and delight wherever they find themselves in life.

Higher activity in the right frontal lobe, however, predisposes a person to the pattern of a melancholic temperament. Those with this condition cannot seem to turn off their pessimism about themselves, others, and life in general. They get hung up on minor problems and are prone to moodiness. Davidson demonstrated that babies who cried when their mothers left the room invariably had more activity in the right frontal lobe than the left. Those who did not cry had more activity in the left frontal lobe.

Here's the upshot of temperament studies for our purposes. Psychological tests have revealed that persons with a cheerful temperament have a lower lifetime risk of depression and other emotional disorders. However, people with timid and fearful temperaments from childhood on develop higher rates of anxiety disorders.

Parenting and childhood experience

So what's a mom or dad to do when raising a child who from birth has a hyperexcitable amygdala or an overactive right temporal lobe (sites in the brain that cause fearful and melancholy feelings)?

The answer lies in providing the right life experiences for the growing child. The wrong experiences — such as any playing into the child's predisposition toward timidity or pessimism — will lead to greater vulnerability and to psychological problems throughout life.

There is a window of opportunity in childhood when the brain is still developing, during which experiences can have a lifelong impact through the sculpting of neural pathways. Some parents take advantage of this window. As a result, about one third of infants born with the timid temperament have lost their timidity by kindergarten. Observation of childrearing practices in the homes of these children show that parents, especially mothers, play a pivotal role. Overprotective mothers who try to insulate their highly reactive and timid infants from anxiety and frustration make these problems worse in the long run, increasing the tendency toward anxiety. The 'best-of-intentions" protective strategy on the part of the parent backfires because it does not allow the timid toddlers to achieve for themselves some small degree of control and mastery over their feelings of fear. Instead, the timid youngster learns that "fear rules" and one's only choice is to react to it, not control it. Overprotective parents tend to pick up a timid, fussy infant more quickly and hold it longer. They tend to be more lenient after the first year of their child's life and indirect or hesitant in setting limits.

The analogy from Chapter 2 of the housebound anxiety sufferer applies here. By backing away from personal management of even the smallest fear-inducing situations outside the home, the person eventually paints him- or herself into an increasingly smaller corner. Similarly, the overprotected child has had every growth experience denied to him or her. A parent steps in to deal with playmate conflicts, choosing clothes to suit the weather, and all the other life encounters that lead a child to conclude either "I can" or "I can't." The child ends up emotionally housebound, unable to deal on his own with most of what life brings his way.

Parents who were successful in reducing their infant's tendency toward fearfulness adopted a "learn to adapt" strategy. They allowed the growing infant to face fears in small increments, while remaining nearby to offer encouragement and support. They do not rush to pick up the child over every little upset or hover to prevent those upsets from happening. Instead, they allow the baby — and then the child — to gradually learn how to manage fear-arousing situations on his own.

Kagan found that parents who put gentle pressure on their timid kids to be more outgoing are most successful in helping their children overcome their timidity. What matters most in determining a child's success in overcoming timidity is his or her degree of social skills. If shy children develop the basic social skills to get along with other children in their first years, they are much more likely to shed their natural inhibitions and develop close friendships. By contrast, shy kids who do not experience social success become overly sensitive to criticism, quick to anger, mistrustful, fearful, and sulky.

So, the headline of the temperament versus life experiences story is this: We can change the influence of the temperaments we were born with, if the right early childhood experiences help to reshape the maturing brain in a positive way. And we have time to do so. Fortunately, the emotional centers of the brain take the longest to develop and mature. Brain development happens in these approximate stages. First, in early childhood, the sensory areas of the brain mature so that we can sense and experience the world around us. Next, the limbic system, which controls basic emotional reaction and response, matures by puberty. The frontal lobes, seat of emotional control, understanding, and thoughtful response, continue to develop into young adulthood.

During this development process — and especially during childhood — the brain is constantly involved in "pruning" neural connections that are less used and strengthening connections that are more used. If neural pathways that carry signals of alarm and anxiety are frequently triggered, those pathways will be reinforced and strengthened. Anxious responses will become "a habit of the mind."

The human mind is at all times a work in progress, changing its structural nature to respond to new learning (including the reading of this book). Repetition, like practicing a musical instrument, strengthens neural pathways and synaptic connections in the brain. What at first feels strange and difficult can, with repetition, become second nature. For example, in a sport such as tennis or golf, it's important to learn proper technique from the start. The brain establishes the pathways that make up your game and then begins to strengthen them. If these pathways aren't set up well in the first place, we spend years "unlearning" bad habits and relearning good form.

Our emotional lives are not unlike learning tennis or golf. Early on, we establish brain pathways for certain emotional responses, then repeat those responses throughout our lives. If the pathways are maladaptive to our lives and personal welfare, we must often seek psychotherapy or other counseling in an effort to reconfigure our ways of thinking and feeling.

Much of the relearning we painfully and expensively undertake in adulthood would have been unnecessary if adept parenting had provided for the emotional needs we experienced as growing children. Successful parenting provides a structured, nurturing environment that is neither overly permissive nor overly protective. Discipline is tempered with understanding and compassion. Unsuccessful parenting, on the other hand, often occurs when the parents themselves are emotionally ill. Self-absorbed by their own issues and problems, they either neglect or ignore the child's signs of distress. Or they react with fierce, unpredictable, and sporadic discipline, yelling, and physical violence to "show those kids who's boss" and "put them in their place."

We've seen in this section on temperament that some children are vulnerable to later emotional ills from their earliest days. But the key point is that parents can *act* supportively to help their initially timid or melancholic offspring escape the tyranny of their genetic inheritance.

Stress

Defining stress for modern readers is unnecessary. Without thinking hard, we could each list a handful of stressors, both large and small, in our personal and professional lives. Even a stress-free environment soon seems to involve the stress of boredom and ennui!

But here's the question: How does stress play a part in anxiety, panic, and depression? Clearly, there is not a one-to-one relationship between a particular stress and any one of these emotional disorders. Stress that one person cannot endure for even an hour may be endured, even enjoyed, by another person for months or years.

Stress is best viewed as one of the common forces that pulls the trigger of the already loaded gun of anxiety, panic, and depression. As we have seen in our discussion of genetic factors and temperament, the "gun" of our vulnerability to anxiety, panic, and depression may be ready to fire from childhood years on. If, when, and how it goes "off" may well depend upon the stresses we face and how we deal with those stresses.

Freud believed that stress in adult life activates an underlying anxiety or depressive disorder for which we are made susceptible by forces largely beyond our control (genetics, temperament, and upbringing). Kendler refined this position by endeavoring to show that different kinds of stress can tip emotional balance toward different forms of distress. In 1993, G.W. Brown postulated that stress that threatens possible loss and danger (for example, learning of a serious illness) triggers anxiety disorder in some people, while stress that involves actual loss (for example, the death of a loved one) triggers depression in some people.

The message for all of us appears clear: Learn to recognize, monitor, and — to the greatest extent possible — control the stresses in our lives. In the following categories of stresses, our goal is to alert you to areas of stress you may be experiencing but may not be recognizing at a conscious level or making an effort to deal with constructively.

External stress

Strictly defined, no stress is truly external. Stress, after all, is our internal response to situations. Things on the "outside" aren't stressful for us...until we make them so. Is sunshine stressful? Certainly not for the surfer waiting for the next, great wave. However, it certainly is for the person worrying about getting skin cancer.

However, for our purposes external stresses will be considered all those events, people, circumstances, desires, needs, obligations, and situations having their point of origin "outside our skin." They are there usually without our choosing or our ability to control them to any great degree.

Work stress

The list of work stressors could fill this book. Michelle Osborne of the Gannett News Service writes, "the number of workers feeling highly stressed has doubled since 1985 to 46 percent in 1999. Job stress is an epidemic, causing accidents as well as a range of illnesses that cost businesses $300 billion a year in health care costs, absentee-ism, and turnover."

High on the list of work stressors are relations with bosses and/or co-workers. In fact, the most common reason given for leaving a job is not money but, instead, "I couldn't get along with the people there." What is there about a particular boss that makes your neck muscles go into spasm? Why do certain co-workers drive you crazy by their incessant quibbles and squabbles?

With a bit of reflection, you can probably identify quite accu-rately who stresses you out at work and why—at least from your own point of view. Identifying these stress sources is the first step in dealing with them.

Work schedules also produce stress. The Families and Work Institute found in a 1998 survey that the average time we Americans spend at our full-time job has risen during the last several years from 43.6 to 47.1 hours per week. That adds up to an extra four weeks of work per year.

Lunch breaks? They used to be an hour long. Now they are com-monly taken at a "working lunch," sitting at the computer screen— one hand on the keyboard and the other hand on a sandwich or a doughnut.

Work stresses spill over into the home. In four out of five mar-riages, both partners work full time. Many bring work home with them under the banner of "telecommuting" or simply finishing dur-ing the evening or on weekends what couldn't be finished during the workday. Beepers, e-mail, cellular phones, and fax machines bring work to us no matter where we are. Working mothers spend less time with their young children, to the point that many toddlers in the United States now learn the language of their foreign-born caregiver as their first and primary language.

There are personal strains and dislocations from layoffs, downsizings, company mergers, and reorganizations. We may feel that we are treated unfairly at work or are not appreciated. All of this adds to our experience of workplace stress.

Finally, we are understandably stressed by working for more years than we had ever intended. As housing costs and medical costs rise, we feel constrained to hang on to our jobs as long as possible. We worry about losing our medical benefits if we quit. For these reasons and others, the Department of Labor estimates that the number of workers 55 years and older will increase by 6 million by the year 2006.

Work stress becomes all the more insidious when we "buy in" to the very things stimulating our stress responses. For example, not too many years ago, a businessperson's success was measured by how much leisure time he or she had for entertaining, pursuing hobbies, enjoying sports, and family life in general. "She has it made" used to mean that her success level in business exempted her from the daily grind.

This is no more. Success in the new millennium seems to be measured by how driven, networked, and frantic a person is. A cellular phone glued to the ear, a beeper by the nightstand, an airplane ticket to Cincinnati tomorrow and then to New York two days later, several dozen e-mail messages waiting to be answered, and an equal number of voice-mail messages — those are the signs of a successful businessperson today. All take their toll in the form of stress.

Academic stress

We easily underestimate the stress of student life. Besides the turmoil of self-discovery and the social experience, the student is never far from a midterm exam, a term paper, or a class project deadline. The academic requirements, intense competition, and parental expectations all provide reasons for stress — not to mention social acceptance, sports obligations, hangovers, as well as the threat of sexually transmitted diseases.

Students often self-medicate for stress reactions by drinking. In fact, across U.S. campuses, the consumption of alcohol has never been higher on a per-capita basis. By using beer as the crutch to alleviate the crunch during student years, these young men and women establish a pattern that will find them trying to destress their careers by three-martini lunches and after-work drinking binges.

Financial stress

Certain nomadic tribes evaluate a person's wealth solely by how many camels he owns. Being a 12-camel person in that society is a very good thing; being a no-camel person is a very sad and shameful thing indeed.

We have our camels as well, though by different names. In *Luxury Fever: Why Money Fails to Satisfy in an Era of Success*, Cornell economist Robert Frank describes how media images set the agenda for what Americans feel they should own and the lifestyle they should pursue. Frank points out that sooner or later, these unrealistic expectations of luxury lead to overwork, worry about financial resources, and credit purchases. We spend our health getting wealth, then we spend our wealth trying to get health. Financially strapped and stressed people come to their doctors with a litany of "breakdown" symptoms: chest pain, insomnia, dizzy spells, ulcers, feelings of suffocation, moodiness, unexplained crying spells, and so forth.

At its worst, financial stress can lead to manic violence. Take the case of the bankrupt stock trader in Georgia who returned to his brokerage and killed a dozen people, or the Palo Alto, California software engineer who killed his wife, his son, and then himself over mounting financial problems.

Relationship stress

"The great majority of mankind," wrote Thoreau, "live lives of quiet desperation." He could just as well have been thinking of modern relationships — including marriage and parenting. There are, of course, the stresses of divorce, unfaithfulness, illness of a loved one, among many others. But eddying around these major emotional whirlpools are hundreds of lesser, petty, but potent stressors that add to our total sum of misery.

These are the "desperation" stressors of which Thoreau writes. We feel desperate about them because we see no apparent solution: the girl with a jealous boyfriend, the man mired in a loveless marriage for the sake of his children, the wife struggling to please a demanding and deeply unhappy husband, the teenager trying to grow up in a home bristling with tension, sarcasm, and hatred among its members.

Sadly, Thoreau points out, our desperation is "quiet." We allow stresses to build to the breaking point — our breaking point, as it often turns out, is in the form of an emotional meltdown. We don't get out of abusive relationships for fear that we will be alone. We don't devote energy to difficult, sustained parenting responsibilities because we just don't believe the kid is worth our effort anymore. We don't tell an interfering relative or in-law to back off because feelings might be hurt.

In short, we endure stress in the mistaken belief that it will go away by itself. It seldom does. Instead, it preys upon our vulnerabilities (detailed earlier in this chapter) and, too often, leaves us anxious, panic stricken, and depressed.

Gender-based stress

Genetic, biologic, and social differences between men and women predispose women to certain kinds of stresses and increases their vulnerability to anxiety and depression. Unipolar depression occurs about twice as often in women as in men and seems to cluster in the years from puberty through childbearing.

Some may ask, "Isn't this difference just a reflection of the fact that women feel more comfortable discussing emotional distress with their doctors than do men? And don't male doctors tend to label women with depression more readily than they do with their male patients?"

Dr. Susan Kornstein, M.D., Director of Women's Psychiatric Services at the Medical College of Virginia Commonwealth University disagrees. "The consistency of findings across cultures and in community as well as clinical samples refutes this theory." She goes on to point out that "biological differences may also differentially predispose women to depression. Differences in brain structure and function, genetic transmission, and hormonal fluctuations across the reproductive cycle have been linked to higher rates of depression in women. Psychosexual factors may also play a role. For example, role stress, victimization, an internalizing coping style, and disadvantaged social status — all may make women more vulnerable to depression."

Gender influences how men and women respond to depression. When depression strikes, women are more likely to have atypical depressive symptoms. While men are likely to lose appetite and weight as depression deepens, women are more likely to have increased appetite and gain weight. Women are also more likely to develop or have secondary psychiatric problems, such as anxiety disorders, eating disorders, and borderline personality disorders. Women are also more likely to see their doctor with other medical illnesses or problems, including migraines, chronic pelvic pain, chronic fatigue syndrome, endometriosis, fibromyalgia, and thyroid disorders. In Dr. Kornstein's view, "women appear to be more sensitive than men to developing a depressive episode following a stressful life event, and they are more likely to have a seasonal pattern to their depression." The premenstrual, postpartum, and perimenopausal times of the reproductive cycle are times when women are vulnerable to developing depression. (Premenstrual refers to a few days to a week before the onset of the menstrual period. Postpartum refers to days to weeks — up to three months — following the birth of a baby. Periomenopausal refers to months to years before complete cessation of menstrual periods.)

Because of highly positive cultural attitudes surrounding the topic of pregnancy, women's depression during that time is often overlooked. Jerrold Rosenbaum, M.D., writes in the *Journal of Clinical Psychiatry* (June, 1999), "Clinicians have tended to underestimate the potential impact of depression itself on health care during pregnancy, in terms of postpartum depression and maternal/infant bonding. It's hard to quantify that impact, but it is negative." The stresses associated with abortions, miscarriages, or infertility also puts a woman at risk for depression. Finally, a woman's stresses also include powerful psychosocial factors — sexual abuse in relationships; role strain as wife, mother, employee, daughter, lover, etc.; and harassment in the workplace. In many marriages, the woman also takes on primary responsibility (and subsequent stress) as bookkeeper, chauffeur, soccer mom, den mother, main correspondent with friends and relatives, planner of family social events and vacations, and on and on. This complicated web of tasks has been called "the second shift" in Arlie Hofschild's book, *Second Shift: Working Parents and the Revolution at Home* (New York: Viking, 1989).

Another uncharted form of harassment in the workplace are threatening or nagging calls several times a day from a controlling and insecure husband or boyfriend. This person doesn't care if his partner gets fired—her career poses a threat to him from the beginning. Nor does the woman have easy options to handle this kind of harassment. In one study, one-third of the women who reported the calls and sought help from their employers ended up losing their jobs. Only 12 percent of CEOs surveyed thought that employers should be dealing with such "domestic" issues.

Trauma

The variety of traumatic life events that can be significant stressors has already been summarized in our discussion of posttraumatic stress disorder (page 31). The severity of the stress depends on the nature of the trauma, the victim's physical proximity to it, and the victim's subjective degree of response to the incident. A personal assault that threatens life and temporarily renders the victim helpless (such as rape, torture, or kidnapping) may be expected to cause deeper emotional scars than attacks that are witnessed and don't threaten the observer's life.

Age of occurrence is an important factor in determining long-term dysfunction and damage. A child who is sexually molested by a trusted adult will likely carry lifetime emotional difficulties and problems with trust, sex, intimate relationships, and self-esteem. Early traumatic experience can block the normal development of coping skills, as well as the social and emotional growth necessary for eventual confidence as an adolescent and adult.

The sensitivity and temperament of the individual also plays a role in how stress is processed and perceived. Some of us habitually blame ourselves when something bad happens, while others are able to keep their sense of self-worth intact and realize that miserable things sometimes happen to good people for no apparent reason.

Internal stress

We are all subject to stress from sources "inside our skin." These internal vulnerabilities may come from genetic or temperament predispositions, from problems we create for ourselves by unproductive ways of thinking and feeling, and from physical disease.

Personality disorders and the development of depression and anxiety

Some people seem to sabotage any chance of a happy life because their own personality just won't allow it. For thousands of years, humans have tried to find explanations for why people have such different personalities regardless of sex, race, or age. Astrologers have turned to the stars and have explained personality differences on the alignment of stars and planets during the period of a person's intrauterine development and birth ("It's because you're a Virgo"). As we have seen, genetic traits, temperament differences, parenting, social relations, and traumatic experiences can all play a role in shaping personality.

People with personality disorders sometimes make colorful characters, but you probably would not want to live with them. Some are labeled as "neurotic" — the paranoid, histrionic, or avoidant types who are often so worried and obsessed by what might go wrong that they can't enjoy what is going right. They may have the alarmist personality portrayed by Woody Allen in his comedy roles. The alarmist sees the world as fraught with overwhelming problems and lurking dangers. Instead of experiencing life with joy, the alarmist is trapped in a world of "what if's" and "if only's."

Because they make others around them uncomfortable, those with personality disorders often find themselves avoided and isolated. Their relationships crack under the negative influence of self-imposed stress. Their children look for the first chance to get out on their own, and friends and neighbors compete to find unique excuses for avoiding contact. Most people find that life is challenging enough without spending time with those who manufacture stress and feel the need to share it unceasingly.

The person with a personality disorder is particularly vulnerable to anxiety and depression (and can make those whose lives they touch vulnerable as well). Perhaps you'll recognize some of the symptoms of the personality disorders below:

- ❏ **Paranoid personality:** defensive, oversensitive, secretive, suspicious, hyperalert, and limited emotional response.
- ❏ **Schizoid personality:** shy, introverted, withdrawn, and avoids close relationships.
- ❏ **Compulsive personality:** perfectionist, egocentric, indecisive, rigid thought patterns, and a need for control.
- ❏ **Histrionic (hysterical) personality:** dependent, immature, seductive, egocentric, vain, and emotionally up and down.
- ❏ **Schizotypical personality:** superstitious, socially isolated, suspicious, limited interpersonal abilities, and odd patterns of speech.
- ❏ **Narcissistic personality:** exhibitionist, grandiose, preoccupied with power, lacking interest in others, and excessive demands for attention.
- ❏ **Avoidant personality:** fearful of rejection, hyperreactive to failure, and poor self-esteem.
- ❏ **Dependent personality:** passive, overaccepting, unable to make decisions, lacking in confidence, and poor self-esteem.
- ❏ **Passive-aggressive personality:** stubborn, procrastinating, argumentative, sulking, helpless, clinging, and negative toward authority figures.
- ❏ **Antisocial personality:** selfish, callous, promiscuous, impulsive, unable to learn from experience, and often enmeshed in legal problems.
- ❏ **Borderline personality:** impulsive, full of anger, fear and guilt; lacking in self-control and self-fulfillment; involved in unstable, intense interpersonal relationships; more likely to attempt suicide; aggressive in behavior with feelings of emptiness and occasional experiences of psychotic breaks with reality; high drug abuse rate; often co-diagnosed with mood disorders and posttraumatic stress disorder.

Certainly there is hope for patients with personality disorders. But these people must first recognize the existence of a problem and be willing to seek help. Several meetings with a psychiatrist or psychologist may be necessary to establish the diagnosis. Through behavioral therapy, the patient can often unlearn destructive patterns of interaction and achieve much more successful levels of social functioning.

Race and sexual orientation

Underrepresented minorities and the poor are under additional stresses that lead to an increase in medical and emotional illness. African-Americans, for example, have higher rates of hypertension, heart disease, obesity, and stroke than do Caucasians. The stresses that contribute to these conditions are external in part, stemming from the prejudice of others, as well as historical injustice. But the stresses are also internal as these men and women are struggling with issues of self-esteem, providing themselves as role models for their children, and professional skills in an increasing competitive economy.

In addition, a person's underlying sexual orientation may cause stress, especially if the person fails to accept who he or she is, or is rejected by family and friends. Approximately 10 percent of all men are born gay, with a slightly lower percentage for women. These people didn't choose to be gay, nor were they "made gay" by parenting or childhood experience. Homosexuality is part of the normal and natural spectrum of human sexuality. It is not a disorder or illness.

In 1952, the American Psychiatric Association's Diagnostic and Statistical Manual I (DSM-I) listed homosexuality as a "sexual deviation," but explained that homosexuals "are ill primarily in terms of society and of conformity with the prevailing cultural milieu, and not only in terms of personal discomfort and relations with other individuals." By 1968, the Manual listed homosexuality as a personality disorder. In 1980, the Manual removed homosexuality from the list of abnormal deviations and personality disorders, but left the category of "ego-dystonic homosexuality" as a classified disorder reserved for those in whom homosexuality "is unwanted and a persistent source of distress [and]...for whom changing sexual orientations is a persisting concern." In plain language, homosexuality is not a psychological or emotional problem unless the person refuses to accept who he or she is.

Medical problems

Medical illness can directly or indirectly increase vulnerability to anxiety, panic, and depression. The order of distress is often a matter of question: Did the depression lead to physical illness, or did physical illness lead to depression? As we have seen, the symptoms of anxiety, panic, and depression are often identical to those of physical illness. People with headaches, numbness, memory impairment, and dizziness may conclude (with the "help" of the Internet) that they have a brain tumor. People with chest pain, racing heart, shortness of breath, and sweating may be convinced they're having a heart attack. They do not associate these bodily symptoms with emotional illness.

When a patient is faced with a life-threatening tumor or is struck by a near-fatal heart attack, he or she may feel an extraordinary degree of internal stress, leading quickly to emotional instability. A variety of physical ills can trigger anxiety disorders and panic attacks. When a patient seems to have an anxiety or depression disorder, the physician will first rule out medical conditions that may be the cause or a contributing cause. There is no doubt: Those with depression are more likely to become physically ill, and those with physical illness are more likely to become depressed.

Medications and other substances

Several medications are implicated in causing depression and anxiety disorders. Corticosteroids such as prednisone (commonly prescribed for asthma, arthritis, eczema, emphysema, and autoimmune diseases) often affect a person's mood because of hyperstimulation of the system, and, in a delayed way, because of suppression of the body's natural production of adrenaline.

Prescription medications

Blood pressure medications, including beta blockers, methyldopa, guanethidine, and clonidine can cause depressive syndromes.

Heart drugs, such as digitalis, can also cause depression. Patients with Parkinson's disease sometimes experience depression as a side-effect of medications used to treat the illness, such as Levodopa. All stimulants, including amphetamines, diet pills, decongestants, nicotine, and caffeine can cause anxiety during use and depression when these drugs are withdrawn. Alcohol, sedatives like Valium, opiates like morphine and Vicodin, and most psychedelic drugs are depressants (although, paradoxically, these are used in self-treatment to combat depression).

Caffeine

Caffeine intoxication can occur following the ingestion of as little as 100 mg of caffeine per day. To give you a clue on how much caffeine you ingest per day, here is a list of many commonly taken caffeinated products:

- ❑ Six ounces of brewed coffee has 100 mg of caffeine.
- ❑ Six ounces of tea contains 40 mg of caffeine.
- ❑ 12 ounces of soda contains 45 mg of caffeine.
- ❑ Over-the-counter analgesics and cold remedies may contain 25 to 50 mg of caffeine per tablet.
- ❑ Stimulants contain 100 to 200 mg of caffeine per tablet.
- ❑ Weight loss aides contain 75 to 200 mg of caffeine per tablet.

Symptoms of caffeine intoxication include restlessness, nervousness, excitement, insomnia, flushed face, sweating, and gastrointestinal complaints. Doses higher than 250 mg (three or more cups of brewed coffee) can cause more severe symptoms, including muscle twitching, rambling flow of thought and speech, heart palpitations, agitation, and periods of seeming inexhaustibility that later lead to fatigue and depression as the caffeine wears off.

Nicotine

Nicotine is addictive, despite multimillion-dollar advertising by the tobacco industry to the contrary. Although more than 80 percent of those who smoke express a desire to quit, only 35 percent try to stop each year, and only 5 percent are successful if not treated medically.

Many smokers give up social, recreational, and occupational events (as well as air travel) because of restrictions on smoking. Countless others continue to smoke even after being diagnosed with a serious medical condition due to tobacco use (including cancer, emphysema, heart disease, chronic bronchitis, and circulatory failure).

It is clear that emotional disorders predispose one to smoke, probably as a conscious or subconscious form of self-medication. Trying to stop only makes depression and anxiety worse, which is why so many fail in their attempts to quit. The common symptoms of nicotine withdrawal include depressed mood, insomnia, irritability, frustration, anger, anxiety, difficulty concentrating, restlessness, slowed heart rate, increased appetite, and weight gain. It's not surprising that the new drug for smoking cessation called Zyban is in fact an old antidepressant called Wellbutrin. The drug underscores the importance of treating the underlying reason why many smokers began the habit in the first place: depression and anxiety.

Cannabis

Drugs made from the cannabis plant, such as marijuana and hashish, can be smoked, taken orally, or mixed with tea and food. The psychoactive effects are caused by a chemical known as THC. This drug has been used to treat a variety of general medical conditions, including the nausea and vomiting caused by chemotherapy, loss of appetite and weight loss in AIDS patients, and the pain of terminal disease. Those who use cannabis regularly do not develop physiological dependence. However, problems can arise if the individual spends so much time acquiring and using the substance that it interferes with family, school, work, or recreational activities.

Intoxication begins with a "high" feeling, followed by euphoria with inappropriate laughter along with feelings of grandiosity, sedation, lethargy, impairment of short-term memory, difficulty carrying out complex mental processes, impaired judgment, distorted sensory perceptions, impaired muscular coordination, and the sensation that time is passing slowly. Mild forms of depression, anxiety, or irritability are seen in about one-third of individuals who use cannabis.

Alcohol

About 10 percent of adults in the United States are problem drinkers, with implications for lost time at work, disruptions of life activities, increased use of health care, along with medical and psychiatric disorders. Physical symptoms of alcohol abuse include heartburn, stomach pain, easy bruising, fluid retention, headache, diarrhea, insomnia, and fatigue. Many who drink heavily do so to help themselves fall asleep. They don't realize, however, that alcohol also causes early morning awakening and actually decreases the overall sleep time.

The most commonly used screening tool for alcohol abuse is the **CAGE** questionnaire, composed of four questions:

1. Have you every felt that you should **C**ut down on drinking?
2. Have people **A**nnoyed you by criticizing your drinking?
3. Have you ever felt **G**uilty about your drinking?
4. Have you ever taken a drink in the morning (**E**ye-opener) to steady your nerves or get rid of a hangover?

If a person answers yes to two or more of these questions, there is a high likelihood of alcohol abuse.

Designer drugs

Also deserving of brief mention are the "rave drugs" popular with all-night clubs, also known as "underground clubs." A popular example of a designer drug is known simply as "G." So far, this combination of "natural" amino acids has caused 32 deaths and 600 emergency room visits in the United States in the first half of 1999.

Natural, of course, does not mean healthy or harmless. Flooding your brain with a natural chemical can be as dangerous as overloading it with an unnatural chemical. The drug "G" can cause seizures if overused, which can lead to choking and death.

Another readily available "rave drug" is "Special K," known to veterinarians as ketamine and used to sedate farm animals. In humans, it causes a feeling of dissociation from reality, which, like schizophrenia, makes it difficult to differentiate reality from delusion. A hallucinogen, ketamine causes near paralysis when taken in large doses. This is known as the "K-hole," where for several hours, the person cannot move and lies motionless on the floor. Visitors to the "K-hole" have been known to stop breathing when the drug paralyzes their diaphragm muscle. They may even suffocate and die.

"Ecstasy" is yet another popular designer drug. Ecstasy is a combination of speed and mescaline and the use of this drug runs the risk of overheating the brain, causing permanent brain damage. The brain on Ecstasy commonly reaches temperatures exceeding 104 degrees. These high temperatures are maintained for extended periods of time.

Rave drugs can cause permanent nervous system damage, making users vulnerable to psychological problems throughout their lives. Parents, schools, and health professionals must all do their part in steering teenagers and others away from these substances.

Summing up for now

A host of external and internal factors can push us toward depression, especially if an underlying vulnerability for depression exists in the first place. Learning what these factors are is the work of the doctor treating the depression—but it isn't his or her work alone. You, the patient, must do some sustained soul searching and life searching to discover, as best as you can, why depression is pulling you down and holding you back.

Barbara...A.P.D. and Friends

Good friends tell each other just about everything. And that's the problem with A.P.D. How can you tell a friend about the brooding and frightening feelings you're experiencing when you talk with them? "Alice, I think you're a great person but the truth is right now I'm feeling the same kind of panic people feel when they're at the top of the Ferris wheel and it stops." And even if I say that to Alice once, what do I say the next time we're together? Here's the script I imagine:

Alice: "So are you feeling better today?"

Me: "No, I still feel horrible. I wish I was home and away from the stress of trying to be pleasant company. I'm a nervous wreck. Walking from the parking lot to this restaurant for lunch on such a warm day was pure hell for me. I almost didn't make it. I felt waves of panic starting and did everything I could to push them back inside me. It's a little better now that we're sitting here at lunch. But I'm so tired of feeling these awful storms of emotion. Why can't I just be normal like you?"

At this point, I wouldn't blame Alice for politely deciding not to put me on her A list anymore as a friend. It's too much to ask any friend to be your steady therapist or patient listener, especially when the feelings aren't every month or so, but every hour of every day. Those feelings even get boring for me to think about; I can imagine how boring they must become to my friends.

So I avoid social involvement when I can. I "get through" the social interaction I have to endure at work, but I steer things as best I can toward individual assignments and hours alone in my office. Don't misunderstand: I do like people. I wish I could have more fun with them. Instead, I have a repertoire of fake smiles, quick banter, and reasonable-sounding excuses that get me by for most life occasions, but certainly aren't helping me build lasting friendships.

At home? I do love my children and husband. I also know that often I can't be there for them because I'm so tied up by or exhausted with A.P.D. My husband has been wonderful at being the strong one, propping me up and trying his best to understand what's plaguing me. But who props him up? What happens when he hits the wall and yearns for a partner exuding joy and warmth? Do I have to fake those feelings at home just as I fake them at work?

In short, I avoid a lot of people in my life because I don't want to let them down. I feel like I'm the walking wounded, and that they won't willingly want to slow down to help my situation. If I'm sick of thinking about and feeling my problems, why should I expect them to feel any differently?

5 | What's Going on Inside Me?

I f by some sleight of hand you were able to hold your own brain in your hand (do not try this at home), you would probably be underwhelmed. Weighing about two pounds, it would have all the consistency and personality of thick, stringy pudding.

But under the microscope, your admiration for this organ would soon grow to awe. Billions of cells link up in a complex Grand Central Station of control functions, memory banks, perceptual processors, emotional components, and organic equipment for thinking, decision-making, and, perhaps, for spiritual insight.

This is the arena where anxiety, panic, and depression have their genesis and can have the resolution as emotional disorders. For all our poetic language about "heartfelt" feelings and sentiments "from the heart," the brain is where the action is.

Why learn about your brain and its functions? If you've been pointing the finger of accusation or blame at part of yourself (your heart? your courage? your personality?), you may as well point it as accurately as possible. Understanding what may be going amiss at the level of your brain chemistry may exercise an enormous "forgiveness effect" over many other aspects of your body or character that you have been indicting.

In addition, a knowledge of brain structures and chemistry can help you understand the purpose of medications that a physician may prescribe for emotional disorders. The panoply of modern drugs for anxiety, panic, and depression deserve the category "miracle drugs." It's hard to appreciate the miracle if we know more about time slots for our favorite TV shows than the brain's inner workings.

Diving in: How the brain works

Our brain is primarily made up of brain cells called "neurons." Although they sit side by side by the billions, they do not touch physically. For a tiny electrical impulse (for the time being, we'll call it a "message") to pass from one neuron to the next, a chemical substance called a "neurotransmitter" must be present. The neuron that wants to send the message wraps up a bit of neurotransmitter in minuscule bubbles called "vesicles." These are loaded at the end of the sending neuron and shipped over to the head of the receiving neuron.

On that quick journey from sending to receiving neuron, the neurotransmitter material must pass across a space between the neurons known as the "synaptic cleft." At the split second that the message is sent, the vesicles containing the neurotransmitter substance open and dump their load into the synaptic cleft.

Now, the receiving neuron has to do its part. To receive the message being sent in the form of neurotransmitter material poured into the synaptic cleft, the receiving neuron must have the right receptors on its head for all the different varieties of neurotransmitter substance that may be arriving. Scientists have discovered that there are at least seven types of receptors for just one form of neurotransmitter and that each of these types has seven subtypes. With this complicated alphabet, a truly precise dialogue can take place between cells. Multiply these two communicating neurons in this example by the billions present in the brain and you have a glimpse of the complicated "back room" mechanisms underlying thought and emotion.

When the neurotransmitter substance locks onto, or "binds" to, its matching receptor at the head of an adjoining neuron, the electric message gets through. Now that its job is done for the time being, the neurotransmitter substance now falls back into the synaptic cleft. Here it will either be destroyed by the enzyme "monoamine oxidase," or absorbed back into the sending cell to be used again in the future. This absorption is called "reuptake," and is the usual fate of the neurotransmitter substance in the synaptic cleft. The sending cell can send another message as soon as the synaptic cleft is cleared.

The brain chemicals that are most important in the cause and treatment of anxiety, panic, and depression are called "serotonin," "dopamine," "norepinephrine," "acetylcholine," and "gamma-amino-butyric acid (GABA)." For over 30 years, the main theory to explain the biochemical basis of emotional dysfunction has been the "monoamine hypothesis." According to this theory, anxiety, panic, and depression result from imbalances of one or another of three biochemicals known as "monoamines," namely serotonin, norepi-nephrine, and dopamine. Serotonin is the most studied of these neu-rotransmitters. It is ingested in the diet (especially in fruit and nuts) and is also manufactured by the body from an amino acid called tryptophan. (Actually, tryptophan is first converted into another chemical known as 5-hydroxytryptophan [5-HTP] and then into se-rotonin. It's never that simple, is it?)

Only 1 to 2 percent of all the serotonin in our bodies is found in the brain. The chemical was first discovered in 1948 in the bloodstream, and later was found to play a role in the intestinal tract, where it helps peri-staltic motion (muscular waves that move food through the intestine), and in the blood vessels, where it helps in the construction of vessel walls.

Looking at depression as it relates to these chemicals, we believe that depression may be caused by a prolonged deficiency in the amount of serotonin or other monoamine compounds available in the synap-tic cleft. In response, the receptors on the head of the receiving neuron become plentiful (a process called "upregulation") and grab what-ever neurotransmitter substance enters the synaptic cleft. This upregulation phenomenon seems to correlate directly with the onset of depression, as well as some forms of anxiety and panic disorder.

These emotional disturbances improve when the receptors un-dergo "downregulation," or thinning out, as more serotonin and neurotransmitter material is made available in the synaptic cleft through the influence of antidepressant medication.

Here's an example to wrap up this basic idea about the upregulation and downregulation of neuroreceptors. During times of military threat, we increase our military bases (upregulation) around

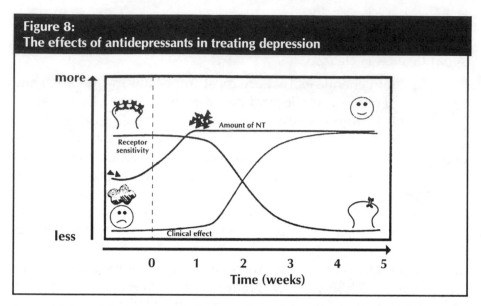

Figure 8:
The effects of antidepressants in treating depression

the world and feel hypervigilant and anxious. During peaceful times, we shut down military installations (downregulation) and enjoy feelings of security and comfort. As in military affairs, wheels turn rather slowly for upregulation and downregulation of receptors in the brain. That's why there's often a lag time of several weeks from the time an antidepressant is taken to the time that symptoms begin to improve.

If your brain's goal is to keep as much neurotransmitter material available as possible in the synaptic cleft, one sure way is to prevent the reuptake of serotonin after it has carried the message from the ending neuron. A class of medications known as "selective serotonin reuptake inhibitors" (SSRIs) do just that. By improving the ability of neurons to communicate, these drugs prove highly useful in treating both anxiety and depression. You may have heard the names of some of the drugs in this category: fluoxetine (Prozac), paroxetine (Paxil), fluvoxamine (Luvox), sertraline (Zoloft), and citalopram (Celexa).

Another class of drugs known as tricyclic antidepressants also acts to block the reuptake mechanism. Drugs in this category include: clomipramine (Anafranil), imipramine (Tofranil), amitryptyline (Elavil), nortriptyline (Pamelor), maprotiline (Ludiomil), amoxapine (Ascendin), and doxepin (Sinequan).

Another way to preserve more neurotransmitter material in the synaptic cleft is to prevent the clean-up chemical, monoamine oxidase,

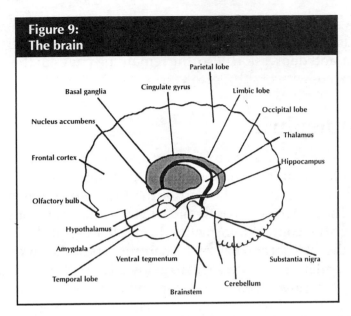

Figure 9:
The brain

from doing its work in destroying the serotonin. This class of drugs, the "monoamine oxidase inhibitors" [MAOIs], are not such household names: phenelzine (Nardil), tranylcypromine (Parnate), isocarboxazid (Marplan), moclobemide (Aurorix), and deprenyl (Selegiline).

The newest medications try to stimulate the release of neurotransmitter substances from the vesicles (those little bubbles at the tail of the sending neuron) or prevent the receptors on the receiving neuron head from taking up too much neurotransmitter material. Drugs here include: venlafaxine (Effexor XR), nefazodone (Serzone), bupropion (Wellbutrin), trazodone (Desyrel), and mirtazapine (Remeron). You can read more about these medications in Chapter 7, "What Are My Treatment Options? (page 109).

Primary neurotransmitter systems in the brain

Dizzy yet with detail? If you are getting weary of chemical compounds, skip ahead to Chapter 6, "What Happens When I Go to the Doctor?" You already have the general idea of what neurotransmitters do in the brain and how antidepressants make them more available to neurons.

However, you may be motivated at this point to go the whole nine yards in grasping the major chemical systems involved in anxiety, panic, and depression. If so, the remaining pages in this chapter are dedicated, with gratitude, to you.

Norepinephrine

The neurons related to this neurotransmitter substance are well located in the brain to handle stressful situations. The center of the norepinephrine system is the part of the brain known as the locus ceruleus. The locus ceruleus is the area that in humans and other mammals receives incoming information from all areas of the body and monitors the internal and external environments of the body. In turn, the locus ceruleus sends messages to many areas within the brain that are known to be involved in the fear and anxiety response, such as the amygdala, hippocampus, hypothalamus, cortex, and spinal cord. It has been shown that electric stimulation of the locus ceruleus in monkeys produces a marked fear response, and that destroying this structure leads to a decrease in the fear response. In short, we have strong evidence that hyperactivity in the norepinephrine system in the locus ceruleus is involved in the development of panic disorder.

Here's how norepinephrine is made by your brain's resident chemist: The neurotransmitter chemical norepinephrine is produced inside a special kind of cell, the noradrenergic neuron. An amino acid, tyrosine (TYR), crosses from the bloodstream across the "blood-brain barrier" and into the brain

Once in the brain, TYR is pumped into the neuron by an "active transport pump," and is acted upon there by three enzymes in succession. First, tyrosine hydroxylase (TOH) determines how much TYR will be acted upon and how quickly. TOH converts TYR into (brace yourself) di-hydroxy-phenylalanine (DOPA). Then the second enzyme, DOPA decarboxylase (DDC), converts DOPA into dopamine (DA). The third enzyme, dopamine beta hydroxylase (DBH), converts DA into norepinephrine (NE). Yikes.

Then the story becomes familiar to us: Like any other neurotransmitter substance, norepinephrine is encapsulated in those tiny bubbles, the vesicles, ready to be released into the synaptic cleft. After

NE has done its job in the synapse cleft, it must be removed before another nerve impulse can be transmitted. Just like other neurotransmitters, it can be accomplished by reuptake (absorbed back into the sending neuron) or destroyed by enzymes. The two main NE destroyers are our old friend monoamine oxidase (MAO) and a new acquaintance, catechol-0-methyl transferase (COMT).

Earlier we attached the approximate terms "sending" and "receiving" to the two neurons involved in the transmission of a nerve impulse. Let's make this language slightly more sophisticated by calling these sending neurons the "presynaptic" neurons and the receiving neurons the "postsynaptic" neuron. Those terms will help us speak accurately about how NE is regulated in the cells and its role in anxiety and panic.

Both the presynaptic and postsynaptic neurons have receptors especially attuned to the presence of NE. The most important of these receptors are identified as alpha 1, alpha 2, and beta 1 adrenergic receptors. What we can observe among these receptors is something akin to an early warning system — NE pours unrestricted into the synaptic cleft. The result, we believe, is one cause of panic attacks. Many chemical clues point to this conclusion. The NE system completes its neurodevelopment by the late teens to early 20s, just the period when onset of panic disorder is most common. Panic symptoms seem to "burn out" as a person ages, and it has been shown that there is an age-related loss of NE neurons that correlates with this reduction of symptoms.

Dopamine

As with norepinephrine, dopamine (DA) is a neurotransmitter substance involved in passing electrical impulses between neurons. Dopamine, too, is made from the amino acid tyrosine (TYR), which is converted to DOPA by TOH, and then to DA by DDC. (If these acronyms start to sound like airport abbreviations, see the chemical names again on the previous page). The same clean-up chemicals, MAO and COMT, destroy spent dopamine in the synaptic cleft. Dopamine has its own reuptake pump on the presynaptic neuron to stop the neuron from firing by sweeping the DA out of the synaptic cleft. There are a host of dopamine receptors, including at least five subtypes (D1-D5).

The most extensively studied of these receptors is D-2. Drugs that stimulate this receptor facilitate the transmission of the dopamine nerve impulse, which is helpful in the treatment of Parkinson's disease. On the other hand, drugs that block the stimulation of the D-2 receptor slow down the transmission of the dopamine nerve impulse. These drugs are used to treat schizophrenia, a disease thought to be caused by overactivity of the dopamine-related neurons.

Serotonin

The serotonin (5HT) system originates primarily from two areas of the brain: the median and dorsal raphe nuclei. These, in turn, have extensive connections with many other brain centers. There is evidence that the 5HT neurons have a restraining effect on areas of the brainstem that are involved in the panic response, such as the periaqueductal gray area. If this restraining influence is interrupted, a panic attack may result. Serotonin is produced in the neuron from the amino acid tryptophan (TRY). This amino acid is converted to 5HTP by the enzyme tryptophan hydroxylase (TRYOH) and then is further converted to 5HT by the enzyme aromatic amino acid decarboxylase (AAADC). 5HT is stored in the presynaptic vesicles until it is released by a neuron impulse. After doing its work in the synaptic cleft, serotonin is destroyed by monoamine oxidase (MAO). The 5HT neuron has a presynaptic reuptake pump called the serotonin transporter. On the presynaptic neuron are the 5HT1A autoreceptors, which detect the presence of 5HT and shut off further activity by pumping serotonin out of the synapse cleft and back into the presynaptic neuron.

Of special importance are three receptors in the NE system. The 5HT1A presynaptic receptor, one of many identified for this neuron, functions as a reuptake pump to sweep serotonin out of the synaptic cleft. Stimulation of this receptor decreases the amount of serotonin available in the synaptic cleft for neurotransmission of impulses. The presynaptic 5HT1D receptor blocks the release of serotonin when stimulated. Finally, the alpha 2 receptor decreases serotonin activity when a different neurotransmitter, NE (see page 91), binds to it.

The goal, of course, in inhibiting or blocking these receptors is to allow serotonin to build up in the synaptic cleft, facilitating neuron impulse transmission. Drugs that downregulate (inhibit) these receptors, especially the 5HT1A receptor, have proven effective in treating depression, obsessive-compulsive disorder, panic disorder, social phobia, and bulimia nervosa by causing an overall increase in the release of serotonin. In the case of panic disorder, there is evidence from a 1995 study by W. Boyer that drugs (SSRIs) targeting serotonin release may be superior to the standard antipanic drugs, including imipramine and alprazolam.

The benzodiazepine/gamma-aminobutyric acid neuronal system

The brain's major system for slowing things down, inhibiting panic sensations, and allowing relaxation is the gamma-aminobutyric acid (GABA) neuronal system. It is an extensive network of linked neurons capable of modulating and suppressing neuronal excitement throughout the brain. Benzodiazepines are drugs that target the GABA system, binding to the GABA receptors and triggering neuron inhibition. The result is a variety of pharmocological effects, including muscle relaxation, blocking of anxiety, blocking of seizure activity, and sedation. The feeling of suffocation is very common in panic attacks, and the hyperventilation that results causes a variety of physical sensations that make the attack even more uncomfortable. These sensations include dizziness, numbness, tingling, and nausea. Patients with panic disorder show rapid improvement in symptoms after administration of these drugs. Their brand names are almost as familiar as penicillin and aspirin: diazepam (Valium), alprazolam (Xanax), lorazepam (Ativan), clorazepate (Tranxene), and clonazepam (Klonopin).

The amygdala

What's true in rats isn't necessarily true in humans; nevertheless, it is striking that when the amygdala is surgically removed in rats, the fear response is blocked. In humans, the amygdala has strong anatomical connections with the hypothalamus and brainstem regions, which have found to be active in producing many symptoms of fear and anxiety. It is thought that the central nucleus of the amygdala is where learning processes relevant to fear and anxiety occur. When the amygdala neurochemical N-methyl-D-aspartate (NMDA) is blocked, the acquisition of conditioned fear responses is also blocked. The clinical implications of knowing how the brain learns to be afraid are that therapies can be developed aimed at blocking phobic learning or facilitating the extinction of phobic learning. Medications that slow down the NMDA/glutamate system may prevent phobia acquisition or help facilitate the extinction of phobias along with behavior therapies.

EEG studies

The electroencephalogram (EEG) is an apparatus that measures and records brain wave activity. People with panic and anxiety have been found to have differences on their EEGs from people who don't have these disorders. In one study, 30 percent of patients had minor EEG abnormalities, and a large percentage of these patients (61 percent) had abnormalities in their brain scans, especially in the septohippocampal area.

Alpha waves are brain waves known to be important in the relaxation response studied by Herbert Benson, and amplification of alpha waves is the goal of some biofeedback therapies. Panic disorder has been linked to an inherited trait of low-voltage alpha waves seen on the EEG. Alcoholics with anxiety disorders are 10 times more likely to exhibit the low-voltage alpha wave trait than normal controls. This trait has been mapped genetically and found to be located on chromosome 20q of the human genome.

Patients with mood disorders have different EEG changes from those with panic disorder, supporting the biological distinction between the two. Patients with panic disorder don't experience the reduction of rapid eye movement (REM) sleep seen in patients with depression. In addition, sleep panics were found to occur in stage three, non-REM sleep. Because sleep panic is a spontaneous attack, its presence helps confirm the diagnosis of panic disorder.

Cardiovascular physiology and panic

A nearly universal symptom of anxiety and panic is accelerated heartbeat and heart palpitations. Adrenaline release in response to stress may be partly involved. The autonomic nervous system is also thought to play a role. The sympathetic nervous system activates and speeds up the heart rate, and the parasympathetic nervous system slows down the heart rate by way of the vagus nerve. Panic patients have been found to have decreased input from the vagus nerve, which allows a predominance of sympathetic nervous system stimulation of the heart, leading to the pounding and palpitating cardiac symptoms.

Neuroimaging techniques

Neuroimaging studies are performed with a variety of brain scans that are able to show differences in structure between patients known to have emotional illness and healthy control patients. These studies show increased areas of metabolism in those parts of the brain that are stimulated during different emotional states. In other words, areas of the brain that are activated by a particular emotional state will light up on the scan. These studies have shown that frontal, temporal, and limbic/hippocampal areas are triggered in panic disorder patients. The medial frontal cortex and orbitofrontal cortex play a role in limiting fear reactions and in unlearning preprogrammed anxiety responses. The anterior cingulate gyrus is involved in both normal and pathological anxiety states. Neuroimaging has also established the activation of the amygdalocortical system during fear conditioning.

 # Summing up for now

Even with this brief discussion of neurobiology, it becomes clear that our brain neurons have a complex language of neurotransmitters and receptors to allow successful and precise communication between neurons. Interconnections between several brain structures determine how we are "wired." Modern medications and behavioral therapies take advantage of knowing this "brain language" and brain structure to create drug and behavioral treatments designed to manipulate brain function to the advantage of the patient suffering from emotional disorders.

No one would claim that a sufferer from anxiety, panic, or depression must know the chemistry of the brain as a prerequisite to treatment and recovery. But in the same way that a diabetes patient wants and deserves some insight into why insulin is necessary, or a heart patient needs to understand what cholesterol does in the body, so people facing emotional illness feel more in control of their treatment when they begin to understand what drugs and other therapies are intended to do in their systems.

Barbara...A.P.D. and Hypochondria

Maybe one of the most frustrating things about A.P.D. is the abysmal physical sensations that accompany it. It may be "all in my head," but I certainly feel a good portion of it in my body.

Let's say I'm asked to stand up to give a short impromptu talk at work. My stomach lurches as devastating thoughts start to pop like firecrackers in my head: What if I start panicking and everyone notices? Will I have to quit halfway through the talk? Will I scare others and send them fleeing to dial 911? What about my reputation at work? Will people come by my office to ask if I'm okay?

I feel my heart rate rising dramatically. Simply by holding my breath for a second I can feel a couple heartbeats and judge whether I'm at 80, 100, or higher beats per minute. Then, of course, all the heart scares come to mind: How can my heart keep this up?

A palpitation or two (sudden irregular heartbeats) raises the ante of nerves substantially, sending new surges of adrenaline through my already overcharged body. Am I having a heart attack?

All this time, of course, I'm trying to carry on in my talk so that no one observes my stress. All my effort goes into keeping my voice from cracking, keeping my shaky hands out of sight, and not letting perspiration plink off my nose. At this point, I'm getting more and more afraid of the fear symptoms crashing through me. I'm trying to hold back full panic, but I'm not sure I can. I rush to get through the speech.

And I make it through, but my system will rush on for a half hour or more after this fight with A.P.D., and feelings of exhaustion, frustration, and fear for the future will last much longer.

Because I'm so prone to focusing on my physical sensations, I make it a point never to read articles or watch TV shows about strokes, aneurysms, cancer, or anything else that my mind can prey upon. I can imagine, though, how people with A.P.D. gradually add to their collection of physical sensations to worry about. I would pay a fortune to never give these things a second thought again in my life.

6 | What Happens When I Go to the Doctor?

The phrases "self-treatment" and "self-medication" have been used throughout the book thus far in a negative context. You may ask what's wrong with "doing it yourself" when it comes to dealing with anxiety, panic, and depression? Aren't we always telling people to take responsibility for their problems—to "own" their illnesses and take control over them?

Well, yes and no. On one hand, yes: No one ever recovers from anxiety, panic, and depression without personal effort and commitment. It's hard work to change patterns of living, thinking, and feeling. No medication or health professional can do that work for you.

On the other hand, no: A sufferer from emotional illness usually should not invent a self-treatment program, such as taking the edge off uncomfortable feelings with increasing alcohol use, marijuana, or other substances. As it should be apparent from even a casual reading of Chapter 5, "What's Going On Inside Me?" emotional illnesses have complicated causes that require expert help to discover and treat. What's more, symptoms of anxiety, panic, and depression may turn out actually to be indications of a serious physical illness. Guessing wrong through self-diagnosis and self-treatment can be risky indeed.

When to seek professional help

How do you know when it is time to check out your symptoms with a doctor? If you are in the grip of anxiety, panic, or depression, you may not be the best one to answer that question. "There's nothing wrong," the housebound panic sufferer tells relatives and friends. "I feel fine. I'm just too busy with home projects to get out much." The truth, of course, is that the person is desperately sick with panic disorder and needs professional intervention. Similarly, a depression sufferer may literally not get out of bed for days on end, or in a manic stage, may work incessantly without sleeping. In many cases these people will not suddenly say, "Well, I'm sleeping too much. I'd better see the doctor," or "Hmm, I'm feeling much too fantastic and don't seem to need sleep at all. I'd better see the doctor."

You may know full well that something's wrong. Or someone who cares about you — a spouse, friend, relative, or co-worker — will let you know that something's not right. The words they choose to say to you may be indirect: "Linda, you seem really down. Maybe you should see someone." "John, I've never seen you so wired. Is everything okay?" "Richard, you've turned down three business trips that involve flying. It's getting to be a problem."

In short, when symptoms of anxiety, panic, and depression are interfering with your daily life, it's time to see your doctor. Specifically, get professional help now if:

❑ You find it an almost insurmountable struggle on a repeated basis to get out of bed to face the day.

❑ You can't turn off worrisome thoughts long enough to eat regularly and sleep well.

❑ You have lost your appetite and haven't eaten much for days.

❑ You are fearful that some kind of "spell" or "attack" of fearful feelings or physical symptoms will strike you.

❑ You think or speak seriously, casually, or in a frequent joking way about ending your life.

❑ You experience physical symptoms such as headaches, diarrhea, and heart palpitations that get in the way of your daily living, or cause you to compromise your plans.

❏ You find yourself crying unexpectedly at the drop of a thoughtless remark or the passing of a sad thought.
❏ You can't seem to focus and concentrate on work tasks and home matters.
❏ You feel shaky, unable to cope, and stressed to your limit.

It's to be expected that we each have different thresholds for noticing the severity of symptoms. In the words of Andrew Solomon, who chronicles his personal battle with severe depression in "Anatomy of Melancholy" (*New Yorker*, Jan. 12, 1998):

> "Some people are disabled by levels of depression that others can handle, and some contrive to function despite serious symptoms. Antidepressants help those who help themselves. To take medication as part of the battle is to battle fiercely, and to refuse them is as ludicrous as entering a modern war on horseback."

As we shall see in detail, many modes of treatment (including but not limited to antidepressants) are available for anxiety, panic, and depression. We should not be quick to dismiss somewhat non-traditional approaches to treatment, especially when they are accompanied by good common sense that promotes emotional health.

Take, for example, the vastly popular book *Healing Anxiety with Herbs* by Dr. Harold H. Bloomfield. His advice for learning to care for yourself and your emotional health is certainly as valuable, if not more, than anything he proposes about the efficacy of herbs as medication:

> In a hectic world in which change and frenzy seem to be the only constants, you may feel like a car racing out of control down a narrow mountain highway. How are you supposed to enjoy the ride or appreciate the scenery when you're in constant danger of losing your grip and crashing over a cliff? What is all this tension and rushing for? For many, it's to be able to afford a heart attack, divorce, and psychotherapy for their children.

Most of us take on more than it's humanly possible to accomplish in any given day. Handling innumerable chores and crises at home, work, and in transit while also trying to pack in athletics, social activities, and fun, we hardly find time to come up for air. Sooner or later, as we try to cram more and more activities into less and less time, the body rebels. Human beings don't 'suddenly' develop anxiety attacks. By the time anxiety strikes, there have been years of neglected clues to slow down, reexamine priorities, and listen to your body's signals.

Taking action for your health

Where should you turn when anxiety, panic, and depression begin to take over? Of the many sources of professional help available, give particular consideration to simply seeing your trusted family physician. Of course, you may also be well served by a number of specialists, ranging from psychologists to psychiatrists to mental health social workers to religious counselors and relaxation coaches in all their forms. You may not need medication or desire it. You may simply respond positively to someone else's reassurance and support.

By going to your family doctor, however, you give a health professional the chance to see the "big picture" of your physical and emotional state, including any physical conditions or diseases that may be at work in causing your symptoms. Your doctor has access not only to the full range of medications and therapies for physical and emotional problems, but also can be a valuable guide to timely referral if you need to see a specialist.

Make this appointment with the urgency that you would if you had broken a bone or had a bleeding laceration. Left untreated, anxiety, panic, and depression have been shown to increase the chances of having a heart attack, to trigger asthmatic attacks, exacerbate chronic pain, and worsen diabetes control. Even cancer seems to strike more aggressively in those whose immune systems are damaged by prolonged stress and depression. This is said not to frighten you, but instead to motivate you to take symptoms of anxiety, panic, and depression seriously. Only about one in three sufferers ever gets professional attention. Without treatment, anxiety and depression often worsen, interfering with work performance, home life, and general health. These conditions can slowly steal away years of happiness and productivity — irreplaceable years of life.

Don't procrastinate. Face anxiety, panic, and depression head on. You have nothing to lose and your life to gain.

Above all, seek out a medical professional you respect and trust—and someone who, in turn, respects you, who listens with great care and thoroughness to what you have to say. If you are too overwhelmed by your symptoms, as is often the case in depression and some forms of panic, ask a friend or relative to help you get to the doctor's office. Don't say to yourself, "This will all go away in a week or two. I'll be my old self one of these days." The weeks you wait in delaying medical evaluation and appropriate treatment are weeks of unnecessary suffering for you and weeks during which your illness may be taking hold in more serious ways.

In making this appointment, expect good things. Many of the most uncomfortable and disturbing symptoms of anxiety, panic, and depression can be improved quickly with a variety of effective treatments. Just knowing that you are facing your problem and turning the corner toward recovery will be a big relief. Put aside any embarrassment about telling your doctor about obsessive thoughts, odd habits, seemingly irrational phobias, suicidal musings, and the like. Your doctor has heard it all before and will not be appalled or judgmental. Your doctor needs to hear the truth about what you are experiencing inside and out.

At the doctor's office

Good for you—you show up for the appointment on time. Sitting in the waiting room, you can't help but wonder what lies ahead in this medical and emotional evaluation.

Every doctor has his or her own preferred style and procedures. Here, however, is the general process of evaluation used by one of the authors, Dr. Gardner, in his own practice. It suggests the various aspects of your health that your doctor will review in making an eventual diagnosis and recommending treatment for your situation.

The evaluation begins by establishing a comfort level so information and feelings can be shared openly. You will provide the doctor with information about your medical and psychological history either in written form or by conversation. Included in this information gathering will probably be questions about your age, job, education, and marital status. The doctor will ask about your main complaints and ask you to describe in detail the symptoms you're experiencing. The doctor will want to know about past or present medical problems along the way, such as surgeries, medications, hormone therapies, supplements, allergies, adverse reactions to medications, family history of illness, habits involving alcohol, tobacco, drugs, over-the-counter stimulants or herbs, date of the last physical exam and any abnormal results, and names of other physicians or professionals who have been consulted.

Next will come a group of questions known as the "review of systems." These questions are designed to elicit any problems the patient may have forgotten to mention, including weight changes, sleeping problems, heart symptoms, difficulty breathing, stomach or bowel problems, muscle or skeletal pain, and neurological conditions (numbness, tingling, weakness, pain, memory and cognitive difficulties, headaches, and so on).

Often patients have already made a diagnosis and come to the doctor simply for confirmation of what they have already concluded, have heard from a friend, or have learned from books or the Internet. And sometimes patients are right in their diagnosis. But just as often, they are wrong in part or in the whole, with serious implications for their health.

To get a clearer picture of the patient's condition, the doctor may ask them to fill out a psychological questionnaire or inventory such as the HAM or BDI forms shown in this chapter. Toward the end of the initial evaluation, the doctor will probably explain his initial thoughts and may schedule appropriate laboratory or screening tests. The doctor will also ask for a copy of the patient's past medical records. A prescription for specific medical treatment may be given on this initial visit, especially if the patient is acutely suffering with panic attacks or is clinically depressed. Or the doctor may prioritize treatment of symptoms beginning with the most threatening or uncomfortable, such as insomnia or headaches.

A complete physical may be scheduled as soon as possible after the initial visit. By this time, laboratory tests from the first visit will have been carefully reviewed. The doctor will explain the results of these tests to the patient and probably give a copy of the laboratory results to the patient to take home. The physical examination itself begins with observation of vital signs (weight, blood pressure, height, breathing rate, heart rate, and temperature) and then proceeds "top to bottom," looking at the eyes, ears, nose, throat, neck thyroid, heart, lungs, abdomen, back, arms and legs, skin, neurological system, circulatory system, lymphatic system, and, if indicated, the genital and urinary systems.

After the physical, doctor and patient together review what has been learned by putting together all the pertinent information from the health history, questionnaire(s), lab tests, and physical examination. Often, the doctor has sufficient information at this point to make a clear diagnosis and discuss treatment options. However, additional tests may be necessary, such as a heart rhythm monitor, a treadmill test, chest X-ray, abdominal ultrasound, or stomach or bowel imaging studies, just to name a few. The patient may be asked to take time to get an evaluation by a psychologist or psychiatrist. This additional point of professional view can be extremely helpful to the doctor in accurately identifying the problem and clarifying the diagnosis and treatment options.

Summing up for now

At this point the patient can feel satisfied that a thorough, professional evaluation of health status has been accomplished. There's no more midnight guessing, based on slim knowledge, of what illnesses may present, or haphazard searches on the Internet for someone's opinion about the meaning of certain symptoms. The patient can now focus on the real problem and quit wasting emotional energy on problems that don't exist. (To gain further insight on how your doctor may examine you, take a look at the "Hamilton Rating Scale for Depression" on the next two pages.)

Figure 10:
The Hamilton Rating Scale for Depression (HAM-D)

The HAM-D scale is designed for use in assessing the symptoms of patients with depression. Although the scale contains 21 variables, evaluation of the severity of depressive symptoms is based on the patient's score on the first 17 items.

1. Depressed mood (sadness, hopelessness, helplessness, worthlessness)
☐ 0 = Absent.
☐ 1 = These feeling states indicated only on questioning.
☐ 2 = These feeling states are reported verbally.
☐ 3 = Communicates feeling states nonverbally (that is, facial expression, posture, tendency to weep).
☐ 4 = Reports these feeling states in spontaneous verbal and nonverbal communication.

2. Feelings of guilt
☐ 0 = Absent.
☐ 1 = Self-reproach, feels he or she has let people down.
☐ 2 = Ideas of guilt or rumination over past errors or "sinful" deeds.
☐ 3 = Present illness is a punishment; delusions of guilt.
☐ 4 = Hears accusatory or denunciatory voices and/or experiences threatening visual hallucinations.

3. Suicide
☐ 0 = Absent.
☐ 1 = Feels life is not worth living.
☐ 2 = Wishes he or she were dead or has any thoughts of possible death to self.
☐ 3 = Suicidal ideas or gestures.
☐ 4 = Attempts at suicide (any serious attempt rates "4").

4. Insomnia—early
☐ 0 = No difficulty falling asleep.
☐ 1 = Complains of occasional difficulty falling asleep (less than half an hour).
☐ 2 = Complains of nightly difficulty falling asleep.

5. Insomnia—middle
☐ 0 = Absent.
☐ 1 = No difficulty.
☐ 2 = Complains of being restless and disturbed during the night.
☐ 3 = Wakes during the night—getting out of bed rates "2" (except for purposes of going to the bathroom).

6. Insomnia—late
☐ 0 = No difficulty.
☐ 1 = Wakes in early hours of the morning but falls back to sleep.
☐ 2 = Unable to fall asleep again if he or she gets out of bed.

7. Work and activities
☐ 0 = No difficulty.
☐ 1 = Thoughts and feelings of incapacity; fatigue or weakness related to activities, work, or hobbies.
☐ 2 = Loss of interest in activity, hobbies, or work—either directly reported by patient or indirectly in listlessness, indecision, and vacillation (feels he or she has to push self to work or for activities).
☐ 3 = Decrease in actual time spent in activities or decrease of productivity.
☐ 4 = Stopped working because of illness.

8. Retardation (slowness of thought and speech; impaired ability to concentrate; decreased motor activity)
☐ 0 = Normal speech and thought.
☐ 1 = Slight retardation.
☐ 2 = Obvious retardation.
☐ 3 = Very difficult.
☐ 4 = Complete stupor.

9. Agitation
☐ 0 = None.
☐ 1 = Fidgetiness.
☐ 2 = "Playing with" hands, hair, etc.
☐ 3 = Moving about, can't sit still.
☐ 4 = Hand wringing, nail biting, hair pulling, lip biting.

Figure 10:
The Hamilton Rating Scale for Depression (HAM-D), continued

10. Anxiety—psychic
☐ 0 = No difficulty.
☐ 1 = Subjective tension and irritability.
☐ 2 = Worries about minor matters.
☐ 3 = Apprehensive attitude apparent in face or speech.
☐ 4 = Fears expressed without questioning.

11. Anxiety—Somatic (physiological forms of anxiety, such as: gastrointestinal [dry mouth, flatulence, indigestion, diarrhea, cramps, belching], cardiovascular [palpitations, headaches], respiratory [hyperventilation, sighing], urination frequency, and sweating)
☐ 0 = Absent.
☐ 1 = Mild.
☐ 2 = Moderate.
☐ 3 = Severe.
☐ 4 = Incapacitating.

12. Somatic symptoms—gastrointestinal
☐ 0 = None.
☐ 1 = Loss of appetite, but eating; heavy feelings in abdomen.
☐ 2 = Difficulty eating without urging; requests or requires laxatives or medication for bowels or medication for GI symptoms.

13. Somatic symptoms—general
☐ 0 = None.
☐ 1 = Heaviness in limbs, back of head; backache, headache, muscle ache; loss of energy and fatigue.
☐ 2 = Any clear-cut symptoms rate "2."

14. Genital symptoms (such as loss of libido or menstrual disturbances)
☐ 0 = Absent.
☐ 1 = Mild.
☐ 2 = Severe.

15. Hypochondria
☐ 0 = Not present.
☐ 1 = Self-absorption (bodily).
☐ 2 = Preoccupation with health.
☐ 3 = Frequent complaints, requests for help, etc.
☐ 4 = Hypochondriacal delusions.

16. Weight loss
☐ 0 = No weight loss.
☐ 1 = Slight or doubtful weight loss.
☐ 2 = Obvious or severe weight loss.

17. Insight
☐ 0 = Acknowledges being depressed and ill.
☐ 1 = Acknowledges illness but attributes cause to bad food, climate, overwork, virus, need for rest, and so forth.
☐ 2 = Denies being ill at all.

18. Diurnal variation
☐ 0 = No variation.
☐ 1 = Mild: doubtful or slight variation.
☐ 2 = Severe: clear or marked variation.

19. Depersonalization and derealization (feelings of unreality, nihilistic ideas)
☐ 0 = Absent.
☐ 1 = Mild.
☐ 2 = Moderate.
☐ 3 = Severe.
☐ 4 = Incapacitating.

20. Paranoid symptoms
☐ 0 = None.
☐ 1 = Suspicious.
☐ 2 = Ideas of reference.
☐ 3 = Delusions of reference and persecution.
☐ 4 = Paranoid hallucinations.

21. Obsessive-compulsive symptoms
☐ 0 = Absent.
☐ 1 = Mild.
☐ 2 = Severe.

Source: Hamilton M. A rating scale for depression. *J Neurol Neurosurg Psychiatry.* 1960;23:56-62.

*Barbara...*A.P.D. and Home Sweet Home

I've read about A.P.D. sufferers who become homebound. Although I'm not homebound, I understand how they got there.

Here's what I think goes on: Home for A.P.D. sufferers is the place where you rest up and get it back together between anxiety and panic attacks. Home is where things are predictable. There are no sudden stresses, no requests you can't postpone, no unfamiliar people to worry about or attempt to please. For some people, "home" by this description may be just one room within their house, perhaps only their bedroom.

Home is where you can be away from people who don't understand what you're feeling. And the telephone is nearby in the ultimate case that you have to call 911. The bed, TV, or books are there so you can relax to some degree. You don't have to make excuses or keep up an elaborate facade as you have to at work, church, or elsewhere.

The question, "What if I start feeling panicky and unable to cope? What if my heart starts palpitating?" gets answered in a reassuring way (by you) so long as you're home: "If that happens, I'll lie down, I'll go to the refrigerator and get a cool drink and maybe something to eat. I'll watch TV until 'it' goes away. Maybe I'll even take a hot bath."

But that same question gets answered in a very different way once you step out of the house, even if only to walk the dog, drive to the grocery store, or pick up the kids at school. "What if A.P.D. feelings overwhelm me away from home?" The answers are full of terror and dread: Well, I'll use my cell phone to dial 911. I'll try to pull the car over to a safe spot and sit there working as hard as I can to avoid going into a full-fledged, disabling panic attack. I'll end up scaring my children forever as I sit overcome by visible, unexplained panic. I'll get as far down my grocery list as I can before escaping from the store and struggling my way back to my one safe place, home.

And unless work necessities or responsibilities to family or friends absolutely force me away from home, I could well see spending virtually all my time there. The outside world seems to an A.P.D. sufferer to be full of risk and occasions for panic without help. Home isn't a perfect retreat, but it's better than the alternative.

7 | What Are My Treatment Options?

Whenthediagnosis of an anxiety or depression disorder has been established, a patient will naturally want to know what treatment is best. Of course, treatment options depend on the type and degree of the illness and dysfunction. This chapter will focus primarily on treatment making use of a variety of drugs. Later chapters will explore other treatment options.

The worst option: ignoring treatment

The cost of not recognizing and intervening weighs greatly on the individuals involved, their families, and society itself. Fifteen percent of those suffering from depression will commit suicide if not adequately treated. In fact, on July 28, 1999, Surgeon General David Satcher urged a national strategy for suicide prevention. The eighth-leading cause of death in the United States, suicide accounted for nearly 40,000 deaths in 1998, compared with about 24,000 homicides in the same year.

Apart from suicide, there are many more deaths and illnesses that can be directly attributed to emotional illness. A growing body of literature suggests that depressive and anxiety disorders lead to premature death by worsening the course of many diseases, including stroke and cardiovascular disease. There is strong evidence that depression is a risk factor for developing heart disease in the first place (Penninx et al. 1998). If a patient has a heart attack and becomes depressed, he or she has as much as a five-fold higher death rate from heart complications that a heart-attack patient without depression (Frasure-Smith et al. 1993). The reason for this increase in death rate is thought to be due to an increase in blood coagulation caused by an increase in platelet reactivity, which is known to occur in depression, as well as a depression-related decrease in heart rate variability that may lead to fatal arrhythmias (abnormal heart rhythms).

Consider the emphysema patient who continues to smoke because of depression and anxiety. What about the diabetic who ignores his dietary restrictions and doesn't care if he forgot to take the prescribed medications because of apathy caused by depression?

Emotional disorders aren't just dangerous to those who suffer from them. Bear in mind that when homicides are carried out by depressed individuals, they feel they have nothing to lose. As this book goes to press, yet another horrible story has been spread across the front page of newspapers. This time, it was about a 44-year-old day trader killing nine and injuring 12 of his co-workers, killing his wife and two children, and then himself in an insane act of vengeance and anger. There is no doubt that emotional illness played a part in this tragedy. Recognized in time, it could have been treated — and 12 people would be alive today because of such treatment.

Fortunately, some mental health professionals are now actively seeking out such potential problems before they explode onto the front page. Dr. Bobbi Lambert, Ph.D., is the founder of Confidante, Inc., a San Francisco Bay Area consulting company that evaluates and investigates potentially volatile workplace situations in order to diffuse problems, prevent violence, and reestablish a healthy and harmonious workplace. She prefers to be called in at the first sign that an employee is acting out with threats or aggression, when an initial complaint of sexual harassment is made, or when a workplace romance has gone sour and is upsetting the work environment. Often she is called in too late, and must focus her work on the survivors and the posttraumatic stress caused by a violent outburst. When asked how she explains the meteoric rise in workplace violence, Dr. Lambert comments, "I think it's symptomatic of what we see in the whole culture. Violence has become a more and more acceptable way to voice our frustration. It's also the economy—you read that unemployment is at an all-time low, but there are many people still out of work. And with the advent of technology, there are a lot of older people who are not as employable as they used to be. They don't feel they have options. People used to think they would go to work for a company, be there forever and be taken care of through retirement. That happens less and less today."

She goes on to point out that much workplace violence is really domestic violence no longer confining itself to the four walls of home, but erupting in the streets and on the job.

Those who are a danger to themselves or others need the immediate attention of a mental health expert—preferably in a hospital setting. It may also be the business of the police if the person has made threats to harm others or has made threats or attempts to take his or her own life. If detained for their behavior, a hold is often imposed on such individuals by the law enforcement agency to insure that they get professional evaluation and care before returning to society. In California, this is known as the "5150 hold," which means that such individuals must be admitted to an involuntary, lock-up psychiatric hospital facility until the judge decides they are safe to be released.

As a popular bumper sticker says: "If you think education is expensive, try ignorance." We are just beginning to realize as a society that we pay a much higher price by cleaning up the damage caused by untreated depression and anxiety, rather than dealing with treatment for those disorders. Education and prevention are the only real solutions that we can afford. Surgeon General Satcher, on his unveiling of the national strategy for research and education on suicide prevention, said, "We must reduce the stigma of mental illness that keeps so many people from seeking help that could save their lives. People should not be afraid or ashamed to seek help."

But what about the thousands of people who seek help but are denied by their insurance company? A report issued in July 1999 by the Henry J. Kaiser Family Foundation, showed that nine out of 10 doctors have experienced the denial of a mental health service that they have recommended for a patient by the patient's health insurer.

The study found that denial of coverage for mental health services had the most profound effect on patients' health, with nearly two-thirds of doctors surveyed saying that a treatment denial in the mental health area caused a "somewhat serious" or "very serious" consequence — up to and including suicide."

Tipper Gore, wife of Vice President Al Gore and long-time mental health advocate, has called suicide "a national tragedy and a public health problem demanding national leadership." We are fortunate to have the issue near the center stage in national politics.

For years, many in the medical profession have questioned the misleading distinction that is often made between mental illness and physical illness, as if the two were biologically separate entities. We now know that the mind and body are one integrated unit, and the health of one necessarily and directly affects the health of the other. Although it is true that the brain is the seat of our cognitive and emotional function, it is also true that the brain monitors and directs all body functions directly through nerve impulses, or indirectly by hormonal messages (as described in Chapter 5).

Emotional illness always causes physical symptoms, and physical illness always affects us emotionally. In fact, many physical illnesses, including chronic pain, many autoimmune disorders, and several digestive problems, must address the emotional response to be successfully treated. The mind/body connection has been studied and discussed by a host of thoughtful individuals, including Dr. Herbert Benson in *The Relaxation Response*, Dr. Norman Cousins, Deepak Chopra, and Dr. Jonathan Sloane, among others. At last, medical insurance companies are starting to realize that emotional illness must be treated as aggressively as physical ailments, and that denying coverage for mental illness costs those companies more in the long run.

In 1999, Congress passed the Mental Health Parity Law, making it illegal for insurance companies to treat mental health issues differently than treating physical health issues. In his address to the White House Conference on Mental Health on June 11, 1999, President Clinton asserted, "There should be no artificial dividing line between our afflictions." The conference brought to light the high cost of emotional illness to society. It reported that one in 10 American children have emotional illness, and that only 20 percent of those who need help ever get it. The remainder of these children are at risk for serious dysfunctions — even suicide. In 30 percent of cases where the child is successful in committing suicide (especially in the case of gay teenagers), the parents had no idea that their child was suffering from depression or other emotional disorder.

The time may finally be at hand when there is no longer any stigma associated with mental illness, no more than that associated with back pain, diabetes, arthritis, or any other medical condition. The problem cannot be addressed or improved until all of society recognizes emotional difficulties as common aspects of human existence, just as "normal" in the course of life the aging process or our eventual decay and death.

Which road to take?

The paths to recovery from emotional disorder and a return to health are many. Successful treatment will likely involve a variety of strategies. At the outset, however, the patient must feel a sense of control, self-confidence, and self-esteem in helping to shape the recovery treatment plan. There can be no escape route of blaming others for health care decisions.

Do you know someone or have a relative who wants to be sick? (If not, you may want to read Thomas Mann's classic work, *The Magic Mountain*, which recounts the subtle allure of illness, loss of personal control, and evasion of responsibility.) Perhaps the person you have in mind is looking for an excuse to avoid work and accountability, to get sympathy and be the center of attention. Do they ever get well? They probably don't, simply because they do not want to. Getting well does not serve their interests — at least as they perceive those interests.

Don't let anyone tell you that there is one single, best way to overcome anxiety, panic, or depression. The truth is that a multifaceted approach is most likely to be effective and make the individual resilient against future relapse. Too many times, self-proclaimed "healers" and even some health care professionals take advantage of emotionally vulnerable patients, involving them in a program of interdependence rather than independence. Too many times patients ask the doctor or healer to take control of all decisions regarding their treatment ("Whatever you say—you're the doctor.") Too many times, in the rush to provide services to the masses, the health care profession seems to accept full responsibility for all decisions and take the patient out of the decision-making loop.

This co-opting of power causes patients to feel insecure, as if they can't get along without the doctor nearby to hold their hand. (In some extreme cases, people with anxiety, panic, and depression purchase homes or rent apartments as close as possible to their doctors' offices or the emergency room of a hospital.) Some doctors encourage this mistaken dependence and loyalty, probably unknowingly, for their own ego support.

The best doctor is the one who shows you how to take care of yourself, so you don't need to come back again for the same problem. Unfortunately, the pernicious nature of emotional problems makes a single-visit fix almost impossible. But you get the point: The doctor's job is to empower you to take control of your problem so you can get on to more important things in life. Beware of any physician, homeopath, naturopath, psychiatrist, chiropractor, or any other healer who insists that they know what's best for you, even if you have feelings to the contrary. Their track record in healing others is no excuse for disempowering you. Everyone's situation is unique and requires a unique, self-designed approach to therapy.

The role of patience in treatment

It is most important to remember that there is no magic pill or easy solution to anxiety, panic, or depression. But there are a variety of very effective treatments to consider and try. Here's a good way to think of the work involved in your recovery. Think of your situation as if you have suffered an injury, and a period of rehabilitation and therapy is necessary for recovery—a period, perhaps, of months or years. Give yourself time to consider your options, in consultation with your doctor, and try those things that best suit your personality and circumstances.

Healing can only take place if the brain is allowed to change and find alternative strategies of working. This only happens with experience. With time, experience actually causes change in brain structure by connecting one neuron to the next, either reinforcing certain memories or developing better, alternative pathways to former abnormal or pathogenic brain responses. We can learn new strategies for coping with stress and anxiety or unlearn neurotic and unhelpful responses.

The brain is probably the only organ that never completes the process of development, remaining flexible and malleable throughout life. The more you use your brain, the more it establishes connections and facilitates communication between neurons. For example, on July 15, 1999, many large-city newspapers ran the story about a 15-year-old girl who had the entire left half of her brain removed to save her life from Rasmussen's syndrome, a rare disease that eats away at brain tissue. After the operation, the doctors felt that she would be able to "live a quite normal life," as the right side of the brain could be taught to take over most of the functions lost by the removal of the left, including speech and fine motor movements.

Other evidence that the brain is capable of growth and development throughout life comes from a recent study of the brain of Albert Einstein. A team of neuroscientists led by Dr. Sandra F. Witelson at the University of Ontario published their findings on Einstein's brain in the June 19, 1999, issue of the medical journal, *The Lancet*. They found that the physicist's brain, in a region called the inferior parietal lobe, was 15 percent bigger than the average brain. This region, it has been found, is involved in processing mathematical thought, three-dimensional visualization, spatial relationships, and other mental processes.

Einstein's brain was willed to Dr. Thomas Harvey at Princeton University, and for years sat in a bottle of formaldehyde in a cardboard box behind the beer cooler in the pathologist's office. It had already been studied extensively, and it was known that Einstein's brain contained an unusual number of certain brain cells called oligodendroglia, which support and nourish the brain's network of neurons. These cells are stimulated to develop when the brain is actively thinking and making synaptic connections that need to be maintained and supported.

Einstein's brain was special because he *used* it. It grew to the point of being structurally unusual in one part because, through thought and study, he exercised that area of the brain. Learning is an experience that structurally changes the brain in the number of connections made, and the number of support cells that grow to support these connections. In fact, all experiences cause structural changes in the brain (including reading this book).

In short, healing does not take place in a vacuum, but requires experiences that build self-confidence. Sometimes these positive experiences are made impossible because patients are so miserable with self-absorbed suffering that they can't even start the healing process. In these conditions, they usually benefit from a course of medication to provide a calmness and relaxed frame of mind in which positive experiences can take place. Popping a pill in and of itself is not an experience that builds self-confidence. It can only encourage the proper neurochemical environment to allow progress toward healing. Pills are not the only way to reestablish this environment. Often the brain can improve its own neurochemical and receptor balance without medical treatment, as long as the individual is given a safe and supportive environment with proper nutrition, exercise, rest, counseling, and some structure to daily life.

For some people, the desired alternative to pills are natural remedies and supplements, including herbs and vitamins. Be cautious. Patients often tell their doctors, "I only want to take natural products." Herbalists and homeopathic physicians often use the meaningless word "natural" to sell a bill of goods. Whether it is synthesized or distilled from an animal or plant source, an herb, vitamin, or other substance may still be *unnatural* to put in your body. Quite natural substances like marijuana and the heart rhythm drug, digitalis (from the foxglove plant), can have powerful and often negative side effects in the wrong amounts.

Does it make a difference inside your body whether the drug is "naturally" derived or synthesized? Of course it doesn't. However, a pharmaceutically manufactured drug is more likely to be pure, predictable in its effect, and reliable in its dosage. One of Dr. Gardner's patients explained, with some misgivings, that her homeopathic physician had found a natural treatment for her stress. It comes from the extract of a tarantula spider. This extract is then "potentiated" with whale grease. Natural? When does a tarantula mix with the blubber of a whale in nature? Even if these combinations of chemicals did work, they certainly are not natural.

However, the term "natural" does have some validity in herbal medicine, where an extract of the herb contains the entire plant. Proponents of herbal medicine point to the "intelligence" of nature in combining chemicals in a way that reduces side effects and brings out the positive effects of the herb. For example, researchers once thought that the chemical hypericin was the active ingredient in St. John's wort and was totally responsible for the herb's antidepressant effects. But evidence now supports the possibility that other constituents of the herb, such as flavonoids, xanthrones, and quercetin may contribute to alterations in the metabolism of noradrenaline and serotonin in the brain, improving neurotransmitter and receptor functioning. The isolated active ingredient alone would not provide the same efficacy as the whole herb.

A visit to the self-help section of your local bookstore will demonstrate the hard sell of "nature's remedy" or "nature's solution" on the cover. Nature has no known remedy or solution for stress, anxiety, panic, or depression. To present such a theory is simple-minded and misleading. It makes vulnerable people feel that the natural answer is clear and effortless. Treatment comes down to just changing your diet or drinking some herbal tea and you will be healed. The natural approach conveys the message that medical treatment is unhealthy and should be avoided. As a consequence, people may resist proven, effective medical treatment because they have been brainwashed by the misinformation and hype of the natural movement.

Who takes responsibility when these individuals kill themselves because they didn't get on Prozac soon enough or were not hospitalized in the depths of a major depressive episode? Most of what the natural advocates sell is the positive placebo effect. A sugar pill (or, if you prefer, a mixture of tarantula juice and whale grease) will work temporarily somewhere between 20 percent of the time for whatever you tell the person it is supposed to help. An authority figure could say anything: "You will get relief from your headache, lower your blood pressure, clear your sinuses, and ease your arthritis pain." If the patient deeply believes in this promise, the fake pill will work for some people for a limited time.

Envision the following scenario. Take some "completely natural" substance, like the mulch from your lawn mower, and put it into a capsule. Then, tell 100 people they're being given a free sample of a revolutionary, natural, completely safe, fat-burning formula. If it works, tell them, they'll be invited to appear on a television infomercial to share the good news with everyone.

The grass-mulch product will convince at least 20 people out of the 100 that it helped them lose a few belt notches. Your magazine ads can now feature a few "before and after" pictures, and it's time to start taking those credit card orders for your green wonder drug. The public illusion is complete — and completely deceptive.

People sometimes avoid prescribed drugs because they want something natural without any side effects. *Everything* can kill you if you overdo it, including water. In overdoses, many vitamins and supplements prove to be toxic, with symptoms ranging from nausea and vomiting to rashes to heart palpitations. It is specifically not true that herbs and supplements are free of side effects. Certain herbs, such as ephedra and large doses of hypericum (St. John's wort) can cause a state of nervousness and anxiety. Amino acid supplements, such as tyrosine and phenylalanine, while improving energy and helping mood, can also backfire, causing irritability, anxiety, and heart palpitations.

One patient, a serious bodybuilder, complained for weeks of prostate and kidney pains until we finally discovered he was taking large doses of the supplement creatine. His symptoms rapidly resolved after discontinuing this supplement. Another patient developed a disfiguring black skin discoloration behind the neck and under the arms called acanthosis nigrans, which sometimes foretells a serious internal malignancy. We were relieved to find that his was caused by excessive doses of a B-vitamin, niacin. Hormone supplements, like DHEA and pregnenolone, can also induce anxiety in susceptible individuals.

To summarize, there will always be those who make their living off of people's phobias, fears, and through misinformation. Natural sounds safe and nontoxic. It brings to mind images of pastures, streams, and bird song—far removed from the sterile environment of invasive procedures. But taking more of a vitamin or herb than your body can use has only one sure result: more expensive urine.

The most natural of "natural" remedies

If we are truly seeking "natural" aids to healing, we should look to what humans beings do naturally. Here's a list, all of which have proven useful as strategies in overcoming anxiety, panic, and depression:

- ❏ A healthy diet.
- ❏ Exercise.
- ❏ Music.
- ❏ Pet therapy.
- ❏ Laughter.
- ❏ Learning to release anger.
- ❏ Letting go of past disappointments.
- ❏ Breaking away from bonds of self-criticism, living freely and joyfully.

In addition, you can participate in other enriching and restorative experiences, including psychotherapy, hypnotherapy, behavioral therapy, biofeedback, neurolinguistic therapy, holotropic breathing, meditation, and spiritual healing. With regard to this last item, spiritual healing, it is obviously not the function of this book to "sell" a particular vision of spiritual life or a theology for everyone. Nevertheless, we should not underestimate the power of sense of peace, inner renewal, and forward-looking enthusiasm for living that many people are able to find through their spiritual lives, however those are defined. It is impossible not to observe, purely on an empirical basis, that prayer changes people. One prayer in particular seems to apply well to our concerns here:

> Let me not pray to be sheltered from dangers but to be fearless in facing them. Let me not beg for the stilling of my pain but the heart to conquer it. —Rabindranath Tagore

Drug therapy in the treatment of anxiety, panic, and depression

Feeling some second thoughts about putting powerful chemicals into our bodies is quite reasonable. This isn't the 1960s, and we don't play around with the ingestion of various substances to see what hallucinations, highs, and other effects they will produce. When it comes to drug treatment of anxiety, panic, and depression, anxious patients are often apprehensive about drug intervention. They will have excessive fears about medical treatment.

On the day this book went to press, the emergency room at a nearby hospital called to report the nearly successful suicide attempt of a 28-year-old female patient just one day after she had finally agreed to medical treatment for her long-term depression. Rejecting the advice of her counselor and parents, who recognized her fragile emotional health, she withdrew and developed a distrust of anyone suggesting she try medications.

Just a few hours after finally agreeing to an SSRI depression medication (see page 128), she got a break-up call from her long-distance boyfriend and did not have the strength to endure the emotional pain. If she had been able to start treatment a month earlier, she may well have been strong enough to face this setback without feeling overwhelmed and hopeless.

As it turns out, she had experienced several bouts of depression in her life and had never been willing to take medication. Under the influence of depression, she felt anxious and somewhat paranoid about drugs in general. For her, they represented the final, tangible proof that she was being labeled as "crazy" by her family and doctor.

This fear of drug intervention must be dispelled. If depression occurs once, it is a safe bet it will recur. Approximately 60 percent of depressed individuals have recurrences, and 15 to 20 percent of these individuals will be successful in killing themselves if they do not receive adequate treatment. Those with untreated depression and anxiety are also more likely to die early from strokes and cardiovascular disease.

By contrast, 60 to 70 percent of patients with depression have a clear improvement on the first course of treatment with an antidepressant drug. However, let it be said at the outset that drugs are not the whole answer. We often do not see full remission and recovery with drug treatment alone, and some patients continue to have chronic depression.

Effective treatments for depression have been available for almost 40 years. The first drugs discovered were the MAO inhibitors (page 124) and the tricyclic antidepressants. In the last 10 years, a family of drugs that act on serotonin, the SSRIs (page 128), have taken center stage because of their increased safety and tolerability. These newer drugs do not have to be monitored and adjusted as assiduously as previous alternatives, have fewer side effects, and are fairly safe should an overdose occur.

In addition to the serotonin medications, drugs have been introduced that selectively target the norepinephrine system (page 91). By using combinations of drugs, full remission from anxiety, panic, and depression is becoming a more realistic goal.

The Holy Grail of early research was the hope that we would discover the underlying cause of depression by understanding exactly how antidepressant medications worked and observing how people with various diagnoses respond to these drugs. So far, this close matching of drug to symptom has not become a general reality. Treatment often seems to be an experiment for both doctor and patient as we search for a medication or combination thereof that is well tolerated and gives a successful response in a particular individual.

In making an initial choice of antidepressant drugs, doctors have guidance from their own experience, that of their colleagues, and FDA-approved indications for use of these medications. Even then, we often find another antidepressant drug is a better choice. The same individual may respond equally well to two completely different antidepressant drugs.

Data from large-scale studies do not show that any one antidepressant drug is better than another in terms of overall response. This fact makes us wonder whether all antidepressants really work by a common "downstream" mechanism. For instance, we know that it takes several weeks to see the real benefits of improvement in depression and anxiety with all of the modern antidepressant drugs. This delayed effect is in spite of the fact that the increase in neurotransmitter levels caused by these drugs happens very early in treatment. It may be that we are stimulating the brain to change by giving it an abnormally high level of neurotransmitters, thereby triggering a response to decrease the number of receptors on the neuron, a process that occurs several weeks after the initiation of the drug therapy. This downregulation of receptors may occur equally well with any number of antidepressant treatments.

It should be made clear from the outset that any medical treatment, as well as any herbal or supplemental therapy, has the potential for side effects that are unpredictable. Doctors do not have a Star Trek tricorder to wave over the patient's head to reveal neurotransmitter deficiencies. No blood test helps us decide which medication will be most successful.

But this "best guess" approach to deciding on which antidepressant drug to prescribe need not be a cause for apprehension or mistrust on the part of the patient. Antidepressant medications are among the safest classifications of drugs on the planet. They are not addictive, are generally well tolerated, and can be tapered on or off according to the patient's needs and desires. They do not permanently change the brain; their alteration of brain neurotransmitters and receptor ratios is only temporary.

But that temporary, beneficial change can make all the difference for a person with anxiety, panic, or depression. This period of restoration of normal chemical levels in the brain will hopefully allow a person to face problems and begin to find positive solutions. Self-esteem building experiences cannot occur until the person is well enough to stop crying and get out of bed. The ability to face problems successfully requires a good night's sleep, normal eating habits, and freedom from panic attacks and obsessive-compulsive behaviors. Getting on the proper medication only sets the stage for the healing process to begin.

Patients should be reassured by knowing that there is much therapeutic overlap with the modern antidepressant drugs, and many have multiple indications for use in treating both depression and generalized anxiety disorder, social anxiety, panic disorder, and obsessive-compulsive disorder. It is often possible to treat more than one diagnosis with a single agent. Side effects are usually mild and improve with continued use. If fact, unlike most medications, many side effects of anti depressant drugs will actually resolve as the dose of the drug is increased.

Many antidepressant drugs have fairly predictable side effects that can be used to the patient's advantage. For instance, mirtazapine (Remeron) and trazadone (Desyrel) are used at bedtime because of their sedating effects that improve sleep patterns. More energizing drugs, such as fluoxetine (Prozac) and paroxetine (Paxil), are most often taken in the morning to help the depressed patient get out of bed to face the day. If a side effect is unpleasant and not improving for a few days, the drug can be stopped and another tried in its place.

It is not a waste of the patient's time to experiment in this way. Learning what the individual tolerates is useful in finding the most effective medical treatment for that individual.

The information that follows is worded in the language used and understood by your physician in treating anxiety, panic, and depression. From the patient's perspective, "a little knowledge is a dangerous thing," especially if such information is misused as a formula for self-treatment. The relatively technical descriptions and explanations that follow are intended to provide you with additional information and terminology to communicate with your physician as fully and efficiently as possible.

Antidepressants

Doctors follow these general principles for antidepressant treatment:

❑ Start the patient on a single medication.
❑ Try to start with a drug that is well tolerated and begin with a low dose, if possible.
❑ Let the patient know the approximate period of time before a response should be expected and inform the patient of any potential reactions that may occur.

❑ Discuss the patient's symptoms and any side effects of medication at each visit, perhaps weekly.

❑ Allow a full trial of six to eight weeks at the full therapeutic dose before combining or switching drugs.

❑ Reassure the patient that if the side effects of the drug do not improve or go away with continued treatment, or if a drug shows little benefit after the trial period, there are many other possible treatments available.

MAO inhibitors
and tricyclic antidepressants

More than 40 years ago, the first antidepressants were discovered by happenstance. It took many years to understand how these drugs work—by blocking the enzyme monoamine oxidase (MAO) or by inhibiting the reuptake of serotonin and norepinephrine (see page 124). The early antidepressants work as well as the newer drugs, but they are not as safe or well tolerated.

Some baseline chemical terms have to be laid out to discuss differences in antidepressant drugs. Recall the discussion of brain chemistry in Chapter 5: There are two types of monoamine oxidase, A and B. Both destroy norepinephrine (NE) in order to keep the chemicals in balance. MAO inhibitors prevent destruction of NE, thereby allowing it to accumulate in the synapse to facilitate neuronal transmission. To help out, there are three types of MAO inhibitors: irreversible and nonselective inhibitors, reversible inhibitors of MAO A, and selective inhibitors of MAO B.

Reversible inhibitors are inactivated by large accumulations of norepinephrine (NE). This is important because foods that contain the amino acid tyramine cause the release of large amounts of NE. These foods include cheese and wine. With irreversible MAO inhibitors, the NE would accumulate to dangerous levels after eating tyramine-rich foods, causing serious elevations of blood pressure. But with the reversible MAO A inhibitor, high tyramine levels deactivate the inhibitor, allowing the MAO A enzyme to do its job and destroy the excess NE.

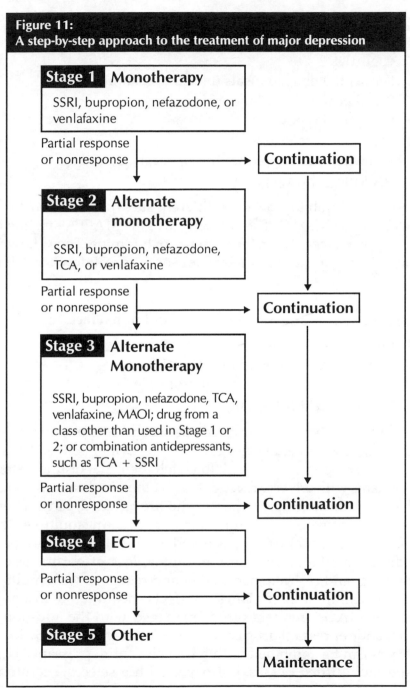

Figure 11:
A step-by-step approach to the treatment of major depression

Stage 1 **Monotherapy**

SSRI, bupropion, nefazodone, or venlafaxine

Partial response or nonresponse → **Continuation**

Stage 2 **Alternate monotherapy**

SSRI, bupropion, nefazodone, TCA, or venlafaxine

Partial response or nonresponse → **Continuation**

Stage 3 **Alternate Monotherapy**

SSRI, bupropion, nefazodone, TCA, venlafaxine, MAOI; drug from a class other than used in Stage 1 or 2; or combination antidepressants, such as TCA + SSRI

Partial response or nonresponse → **Continuation**

Stage 4 **ECT**

Partial response or nonresponse → **Continuation**

Stage 5 **Other**

Maintenance

Source: Crismon ML, Trivedi M, Pigott TA, et al. The Texas Medication Algorithm Project: Report of the Texas Consensus Congerence Panel of Medication Treatment of Major Depressive Disorder. *J Clin Psychiatry.* 1999;60:142-156.

Principal dietary restrictions for patients taking an MAOI include:

- ❑ Cheeses (except cottage cheese, cream cheese, and fresh yogurt).
- ❑ Fermented or aged meats (bologna, salami).
- ❑ Broad bean pods (Chinese bean pods).
- ❑ Liver of all types.
- ❑ Meat and yeast extracts.
- ❑ Red wine, sherry, vermouth, cognac, beer, and ale.
- ❑ Soy sauce, shrimp paste, and sauerkraut.

Selective inhibitors act on a different subtype of the MAO enzyme known as MAO B. These drugs leave the MAO A enzyme intact to destroy excess NE in the presence of tyramine. They allow for overall increase in NE but inhibit some of the breakdown of NE by MAO B.

Classic MAO inhibitors: irreversible and nonselective

- ❑ **phenelzine (Nardil)**.
- ❑ **tranylcypromine (Parnate)**. This drug has amphetamine-like, stimulant properties.
- ❑ **isocarboxazid (Marplan)**.

The drugs above are only used as second-line treatments, after safer and more tolerable drugs have proven ineffective. Patients who are not responsible enough to watch their diet or understand the problems with adverse reactions with other medications should not be given these drugs. Patients who are agitated, have insomnia, have difficulty following directions, or are taking multiple other medications are usually not considered for this class of antidepressant drug. Low blood pressure, insomnia, loss of normal sexual functioning, and restriction with diet and reactions with multiple other medications are the main side effects encountered. Insomnia caused by MAO inhibitors can be managed with the addition of another antidepressant drug called trazadone (see page 138). MAO inhibitors can be combined with a tricyclic antidepressant (TCA) in especially difficult cases, but never with a selective serotonin reuptake inhibitor (SSRI).

Reversible MAO A inhibitors
❏ **moclobemide (Aurorix).** This drug may be better tolerated with fewer dietary restrictions, but is sometimes less effective in the treatment of depression.

Selective MAO B inhibitors
❏ **deprenyl (Selegiline; Eldeplyl).** Even this drug, which is the safest of the MAO inhibitors, should not be combined with an SSRI.

Tricyclic antidepressants (TCAs)

These drugs act on five different receptors in the neuron, a broad range of action that explains both the antidepressant effects of the drugs as well as their many side effects. First, a tricyclic antidepressant binds to the serotonin reuptake pump and blocks it, causing an increase of serotonin in the synapse, beginning to improve depressive symptoms. Second, it binds to the norepinephrine reuptake pump and blocks it as well, increasing NE levels and further resolving the depression. Third, it acts as an anticholinergic and antimuscarinic drug by binding to the acetylcholine receptors. This action causes the commonly experienced side effects of constipation, urinary retention, blurred vision, dry mouth, and drowsiness. Fourth, TCAs block the alpha 1 adrenergic receptors, causing a drop in blood pressure, dizziness, and drowsiness. The fifth effect of TCAs stems from its action in blocking the histamine H1 receptors. This antihistamine effect is responsible for weight gain and even more drowsiness.

Types of tricyclic antidepressants
❏ **clomipramine (Anafranil).** The most potent 5HT reuptake blocker of the TCAs, it also increases norepinephrine. It is effective in treating obsessive-compulsive disorder, but has an increased risk of seizures at high doses.
❏ **imipramine (Tofranil).**
❏ **amitriptyline (Elavil, Endep, Tryptizol, Laroxyl).**
❏ **nortriptyline (Pamelor, Noratren).**
❏ **protriptyline (Vivactil).**

- **maprotiline (Ludiomil).** This norepinephrine selective drug has an increased risk of seizures.
- **amoxapine (Ascendin).** This is a 5HT2 blocker with neuroleptic properties.
- **doxepin (Sinequan, Adapin).**
- **desipramine (Norpramin, Pertofan).** Also norepinephrine selective.
- **trimipramine (Surmontil).**

Even though these drugs are effective at alleviating depression by blocking both serotonin and norepinephrine reuptake, their use is limited by associated side effects due to unwanted pharmacological actions at secondary receptors. TCAs seem to work well for patients with chronic pain, fibromyalgia, premenstrual syndrome, migraine headaches, insomnia and severe depression. Unlike the newer drugs, TCAs can be toxic if overdosed and should not be used if the patient is suicidal. Nor should these drugs be used in those who cannot tolerate the side effects of sedation, constipation, and urinary retention, as well as those who are overweight, have cardiac illness, are demented or senile, or are taking multiple other medications (with risk of drug interaction with TCAs).

The positive attributes of this class of drug include low-cost and significant effectiveness. They work just as well as the modern antidepressants and are possibly more effective in severe depression.

Serotonin selective reuptake inhibitors (SSRIs)

The most commonly prescribed antidepressant drugs worldwide are the serotonin reuptake inhibitors. To call them antidepressant drugs is somewhat of a misnomer, as they have proven just as useful for generalized anxiety and panic disorders, as well as in obsessive-compulsive disorder, and bulimia. They have also been found to be helpful in treating social phobia, posttraumatic stress disorder, premenstrual dysphoric disorder, migraine, dysthymia, chronic fatigue, fibromyalgia, and irritable bowel syndrome among other conditions.

Their main advantage over MAO inhibitors and TCAs is a much-improved safety and tolerability. In addition, they are not lethal in overdose, as are the classic antidepressants. Also absent are bothersome anticholinergic side effects and heart toxicity. Because of these improvements, treatment is better tolerated for those patients who need a long-term medication plan.

On the down side, SSRIs may not work as well as some of the earlier drugs that work nonselectively on more than one neuronal pathway. They also have their own problems, including sexual dysfunction (difficulty reaching orgasm in men and women), sleep disturbance, and, in some cases, increased anxiety. Nausea occurs in 20 to 30 percent of patients and diarrhea in 11 to 18 percent. Headache, insomnia, and agitation are also reported with some frequency. Serious and sometimes fatal reactions have occurred in patients who took an SSRI in combination with an MAO inhibitor or a TCA. Because SSRIs block the metabolic pathway that breaks down TCAs, the blood level of TCA has been observed to rise to extraordinarily high levels, sometimes resulting in heart toxicity.

The main agents in the SSRI class differ in chemical structure, and therefore have very different pharmacological properties and side effects from one another. The major SSRIs on the market in most countries are fluoxetine (Prozac), sertraline (Zoloft), paroxetine (Paxil), fluvoxamine (Luvox/Faverin), and citalopram (Cipramil/Celexa).

In general, SSRIs insert themselves into the neuron's serotonin reuptake pump, thereby blocking its action and causing an increase of serotonin in the synaptic cleft (space between neurons). This increased serotonin facilitates, or disinhibits, neuronal impulses along the serotonin pathways of the brain. The increased serotonin also causes a decrease in the number of autoreceptors on the postsynaptic cell (see page 88). This process takes several weeks to occur, and accounts for the delay in antidepressant effects.

The key serotonin pathways in the brain are facilitated or disinhibited simultaneously by the SSRIs. Understanding these serotonin pathways will explain both the therapeutic and side-effect profiles of the SSRI drugs. Pathway 1 is from the midbrain raphe to the prefrontal cortex. Pathway 2 is from the midbrain raphe to the basal ganglia. Pathway 3 runs from the midbrain raphe to the limbic cortex and hippocampus. Pathway 4 is from the midbrain raphe to the hypothalamus. Finally, pathway 5 runs down the spinal cord from the midbrain raphe.

We believe that the antidepressant effects of SSRIs can be attributed to disinhibition of pathway 1. Improvement in obsessive compulsive disorder comes from disinhibition of pathway 2. Panic disorder is treated by facilitating pathway 3, and bulimia is thought to be helped by disinhibition of pathway 4.

The side effects of SSRIs can be explained as a consequence of the stimulation of the 5HT2 and 5HT3 receptors. For instance, stimulation of 5HT2 receptors in pathway 3, which goes between midbrain and the hippocampus and limbic cortex, can cause anxiety and even occasional panic attacks. However, we already know that disinhibition of this same pathway aids in the improvement of anxiety and panic over time. This effect is due to the downregulation of the receptors that occurs the longer the drug is used.

For this reason, doctors start with a low dose of the SSRI and encourage the patient to continue treatment even if the anxiety slightly worsens for several days. In addition, doctors will often counteract this initial exacerbation of the patient's anxiety by giving some anxiety-blocking medication in the form of a benzodiazepine for a limited time.

Insomnia sometimes occurs with initial use of SSRIs due to stimulation of 5HT2 receptors in the brainstem sleep centers (pathway 5). Stimulation of 5HT2 receptors in pathway 2, which projects to the basal ganglia, can cause agitation and akathisia (a form of muscle restlessness and involuntary movement). Sexual problems caused by SSRIs happen because of an inverse relationship between serotonin and dopamine, with serotonin tending to diminish sexual functioning and dopamine tending to enhance sexual functioning. Because certain brain dopamine systems in the mesolimbic area of the brain are turned down by SSRIs as the serotonin systems are increased, sexual dysfunction results. For this reason, we can use certain stimulants that promote dopamine to counteract the sexual apathy and disinterest caused by SSRIs. Problems with ejaculation and orgasm occur due to disinhibition of pathway 5, which descends from the brainstem down the spinal cord to the spinal reflexes in charge of these activities.

The other side effects of SSRIs are a consequence of 5HT3 stimulation, which causes nausea, diarrhea, abdominal pains, and headaches. The loss of appetite, nausea, and weight loss that often occur with SSRIs may be due to activation (disinhibition) of serotonin pathway 4 from the brainstem to the hypothalamus, an area that regulates appetite and eating behaviors. The abdominal cramps and diarrhea that may be seen with SSRIs are thought to be due to stimulation of 5HT3 receptors located in the wall of the intestines which trigger increased bowel movement.

The generalizations that can be made about the SSRI class of drugs are as follows:

1. There is no way of knowing in advance how well the drug will be tolerated, which of the SSRIs will be best tolerated, how soon the positive response will occur, or what dosage is best for a particular individual. The only way to find out is to be willing to experiment, knowing that minor side effects generally resolve themselves or can be counteracted, and that these drugs are among the safest in modern medicine.

2. Knowing a patient's primary diagnosis and the symptoms caused by that illness can guide the physician in choosing a drug that may be best expected to help without exacerbating the situation. A careful medical and psychological history is therefore crucial before a therapy is initiated.

3. Some feel that the SSRIs are not as powerful as the TCAs for severe depression. However, SSRIs can often be mixed with other drugs to improve effectiveness and decrease side effects, if needed.

4. Sexual dysfunction can be improved in a number of ways. One way is to switch to a drug that blocks the 5HT2 receptor and/or increased norepinephrine and dopamine concentrations in the synapse, such as nefazodone (Serzone), mirtazepine (Remeron), or bupropion (Wellbutrin). Dopamine enhancing agents, such as amantidine, bromocriptine, methylphenidate, and d-amphetamine could also be tried along with the SSRI. Adding Serzone or buspirone (Buspar) has also worked in some individuals.

Here is some additional information and a summary of each of the SSRI drugs.

Fluoxetine (Prozac)

Indications and uses: Patients with major depression, obsessive-compulsive disorder, and bulimia nervosa.

Advantages: It is the only SSRI with FDA approval for bulimia nervosa, has the lowest incidence of sexual dysfunction in the SSRI class, and promotes weight loss that may be helpful to those who overeat during depression.

Disadvantages: The comparatively more common side effects of anxiety, agitation, and insomnia.

Notable drug interactions: When it is taken with buspirone (Buspar), it may paradoxically worsen OCD. It should not be mixed with the TCAs.

Administration and dosage: For depression: Start at 10 to 20 mg/day taken in the morning; it may adjusted to 80 mg/day if needed. For OCD: Start at 10 to 20 mg/day, adjust to 80 mg/day maximum if needed. For bulimia nervosa: Start at 60 mg/day and maintain this dose if it is tolerated.

Availability: 10- and 20-mg capsules, liquid syrup at 20- mg/5-mL dose.

Sertraline (Zoloft)

Indications and uses: Major depression, panic disorder, and OCD in adults and children.

Advantages: FDA approval for use in children.

Disadvantages: Usually, the dose needs to be increased to provide continued effectiveness and the final maintenance dose is usually two to four times the starting dose. Diarrhea is a comparatively more common side effect.

Notable drug interactions: It increases the blood thinning effects of Warfarin, and it should not be given at the same time as a TCA.

Administration and dosage: For depression: Start at 50 mg/day, adjust up to 200 mg/day as needed. For OCD: Start at 25 mg/day for children and 50 mg/day for adults. Maximum dose 200 mg/day. panic disorder: Start at 25mg/day. Maximum dose 200 mg/day.

Availability: Comes in 25-, 50-, and 100-mg scored tablets and capsules.

Paroxetine (Paxil)

Indications and uses: Major depression, OCD, panic disorder, and social phobia.

Advantages: Expanded indications, helpful for mixed depression with anxiety.

Disadvantages: Paxil is not FDA approved for use in children. There are more adverse side effects than seen in other SSRIs, including constipation, dry mouth, and sexual dysfunction.

Notable drug interactions: Cimetidine (Tagamet) increases Paxil concentration by about 50 percent. Phenytoin (Dilantin) reduces the amount of effective Paxil and increases its removal from the body. Paxil should not be used with TCAs.

Administration and dosage: For depression: Start at 20 mg/day, adjust up to 50 mg/day if needed. For OCD: Start at 40 mg/day, adjust down to 20 mg if side effects occur or up to 60 mg/day if needed. For panic disorder: Start at 40 mg/day, adjust down to 10 mg or up to 60 mg/day as indicated.

Availability: Comes in 10-, 20-, 30-, and 40-mg scored tablets, and 20- and 30-mg coated tablets.

Fluvoxamine (Luvox)

Indications and uses: For use in curing OCD in adults and children.

Advantages: Luvox may be used in children.

Disadvantages: Luvox is more expensive and has only one indication for use (OCD). It has the highest reported incidence of nausea and commonly causes sexual dysfunction.

Notable drug interactions: Warfarin (Coumadin) was increased by 98 percent in the blood; Hismanal and Seldane levels are increased to dangerous levels. Luvox should also should be avoided if taking carbamazepine, benzodiazepines, haloperidol, erythromycin, quinidine, and verapamil.

Administration and dosage: For OCD: The adult starting dose 50 mg/day, the initial children's dose is 25 mg at bedtime. It may be adjusted up to 300 mg/day in adults and 200 mg/day in children.

Availability: Fluvoxamine comes in 50-mg scored and 100-mg tablets.

Figure 12: Dosages of the newer antidepressants		
Agents	Unsual dosage (mg/d)	Higher dosage* (mg/d)
Selective serotonin reuptake inhibitors		
Citalopram	20	40-60
Fluoxetine	20	40-80
Paroxetine	20-30	40-60
Sertraline	50-100	150-200
Multiple-receptor antidepressants		
Bupropion	225-300	450
Mirtazapine	15	45
Nefazodone	300-400	600
Venlafaxine	150-225	450
*If needed for efficacy.		

Source: *Patient Care* magazine, August 15, 1999; p. 195

Citalopram (Celexa)

Indications and uses: Moderate to severe depression in adults.

Advantages: Fewer side effects and drug interactions compared to other SSRIs. Faster onset of action than other SSRIs. Cost effective.

Disadvantages: Comparatively more vomiting.

Notable drug interactions: Metoprolol, macrolide antibiotics, azole antifungals.

Administration and dosage: Start at 20 mg/day, adjust up to 60mg/day if needed. Don't go over 30mg/day in the elderly or in those with liver disease.

Availability: Comes in 20- and 40-mg tablets.

Norepinephrine reuptake inhibitors (NRIs)

Norepinephrine reuptake inhibitors (NRIs) and the new selective norepinephrine reuptake inhibitor, reboxetine, work by increasing the norepinephrine (NE) available within the neuronal synapse just as SSRIs increase the amount of serotonin: by blocking the pump that removes the neurotransmitter from the synapse.

Norepinephrine was first discovered more than 100 years ago in extracts from the adrenal glands and was recognized as a key neurotransmitter in the body's involuntary sympathetic nervous system. By the 1950s, it was recognized that norepinephrine also exists within the brain, especially the brainstem and cerebral cortex. Astute observers noted the mood-elevating effects of stimulants known to increase activity of the NE system, such as amphetamines and cocaine, as well as the mood-lowering effects of drugs that block the NE system, such as the blood pressure drug reserpine.

Studies have suggested that problems with regulation of the brain's NE system can trigger the body's alarm system, which is thought to underlie panic attacks. This action occurs especially in the locus ceruleus, where agents that increase the activity of the region tend to provoke panic.

Therefore, one would predict that taking a drug that stimulates this system, as do the NRIs, would be like "pressing the panic button." We think, however, that these drugs do not act simply by increasing NE over time, but that they also cause a homeostatic or adaptive response that causes an out-of-balance system to re-regulate itself. In essence, we are trying to accomplish a healing process in using a very old homeopathic philosophy: If you trigger the symptoms of the disorder very subtly, the body will respond by correcting the underlying abnormality.

At present, there is much discussion about the useful roles of NRIs, especially in relation to the TCA and SSRI drugs. The TCAs block many receptors, including the alpha1 adrenergic receptors, which produces dizziness, drop in blood pressure, and accelerated heart rate — a bad combination for the elderly. TCAs also block histamine receptors, which can produce weight gain, drowsiness, and sedation. The muscarinic cholinergic receptor blockade due to TCAs causes dry mouth, blurred vision, constipation, and urinary retention.

The SSRIs are better tolerated, but have a high degree of sexual dysfunction. Since long-term treatment is necessary for many, long-term tolerability is an important consideration. NE selective drugs may prove to be more efficacious and better tolerated than previous antidepressant drugs for some people. Despite its many side effects, the NE selective TCA drug, nortryptiline, was found to be three to five times more effective for treating depression in the elderly than the SSRI fluoxetine.

Patients with bipolar disorder are especially vulnerable to NE malfunction, which may be why they seem to do better on drugs which influence this system. Episodes of mania may still need to be controlled by adding a mood stabilizing drug, which will be discussed later in this section on drug treatment.

Panic disorder, as well as GAD, social phobia, and OCD have all been effectively treated by the SSRIs. In the past, TCAs were used to treat panic disorders, particularly TCAs that target the NE system. Desipramine, a relatively pure NRI, has been shown to be better at treating panic than the other TCAs.

The newest drug, reboxetine, is the first in a class of selective NE reuptake inhibitors. These newer drugs target the NE system selectively, eliminating the bothersome side effects of the TCAs. Reboxetine and its cousins may finally give us better long-term control and tolerability in depression and anxiety disorders.

Selective drugs for other neurotransmitter mechanisms

The list of modern-day antidepressants includes a number of drugs that have mechanisms of action on the brain's neurotransmitter system quite different from the MAOIs, TCAs, SSRIs, and NRIs discussed so far. Here's a summary of these drugs:

Venlafaxine (Effexor XR)

Mechanism of action: Blocks both serotonin and norepinephrine reuptake and possibly also blocks dopamine reuptake. Sometimes called a "broad spectrum" antidepressant, this drug kept the SSRI and NRI pharmacological effects of the TCAs, but got rid of the alpha 1, antihistamine, and muscarinic anticholinergic properties to create a better-tolerated and perhaps more effective drug. Serotonin reuptake is inhibited at low doses, and the drug behaves essentially the same as an SSRI. At medium doses, the NE reuptake inhibition occurs, improving symptoms of melancholia and severe depression. The dopamine reuptake blockade happens only at higher doses.

Indications and uses: Major depression (adults) and general anxiety disorder.

Advantages: The antidepressant effect occurs rapidly with improvement in attention, concentration, memory, and coordination. It is useful in depressive patients who tend to gain weight, oversleep, have slow movement, and diminished mental abilities. There is a low likelihood of drug interactions other than with the MAOIs.

Disadvantages: At a low dose, it can cause the same side effects as SSRIs, including nausea, agitation, sexual dysfunction, and insomnia. At medium to high doses, the NE and dopamine effects may cause increased blood pressure, insomnia, nausea, and headache. Trazadone at bedtime is often added to counteract the insomnia. Mirtazapine (Remeron) may be useful for the nausea, insomnia, and agitation. Venlafaxine commonly has withdrawal effects if discontinued suddenly, including nausea, diarrhea, dizziness, and sweating.

Notable drug interactions: MAOIs and Cimetidine.

Administration and dosage: 37.5 to 150 mg/day in one dose. Can be given in doses up to 300 mg/day in one dose. At doses under 150 mg/day, this drug acts much like a SSRI. Only at doses over 150 mg do the norepinephrine effects appear. In this regard, it is really two different drugs. These is no benefit to the short-acting form of Effexor, and only the XR (extended release, once a day) form of the drug should be used.

Availability: 37.5-, 75-, and 150-mg doses.

Nefazadone (Serzone)

Mechanism of action: Nefazadone acts by blocking the serotonin 5HT2 receptor (unlike SSRIs that stimulate the 5HT2 receptor), coupled with less-powerful serotonin and norepinephrine reuptake blockade.

Indications and uses: Adult patients with major depression associated with anxiety.

Advantages: Blockade of the 5HT2 receptor reduces anxiety, enhances deep sleep, and causes no sexual dysfunction, but can be sedating. In the short term, it reduces anxiety and insomnia unlike the SSRIs which may exacerbate these conditions.

Disadvantages: The sedation and inhibition of the P450 metabolic pathway which breaks down many medications in the liver that gives nefazadone the potential for drug interactions.

Notable drug interactions: Seldane (taken off the market) and Hismanal (no longer available in the United States) and Propulcid can all cause serious heart rhythm problems if mixed with Nefazadone. Four percent of Caucasians lack the enzyme to metabolize nefazadone, causing an immediate agitation, a flu-like syndrome, dizziness, nausea, and insomnia.

Administration and dosage: Initial dose: 100 mg, twice a day. Dose range of 300 to 600 mg/day in a divided dose. In the elderly, consider all dosing once daily at night. For elderly patients with dementia or agitated depression, consider nefazadone in the morning with trazadone at bedtime.

Dr. Michael Gitlin, M.D., Professor of Psychiatry at UCLA, believes that Serzone is best given as a single dose at bedtime, up to 600 mg, to minimize side effects and increase compliance with a simpler, once-a-day dosing. At low doses, Serzone is a good sedative. Effective treatment of depression, however, according to Dr. Gitlin, requires doses in the 450-600 mg/day range.

Availability: 100-, 200-, and 250-mg tablets.

Trazadone (Desyrel)

Mechanism of action: Serotonin 5HT2 blocker and serotonin reuptake blocker, with strong histamine and alpha 1 blockade. There is no NE activity.

Indications and uses: Depression and anxiety, especially with insomnia.

Advantages: Sedating effects of histamine receptor blockade.

Disadvantages: Nefazadone is a better antidepressant with less sedating effects.

Drug interactions: Same as nefazadone.

Administration and dosage: Initial dose: 50 mg at bedtime. It may be increased to as much as 200 mg at bedtime.

Availability: Comes in 50- and 150-mg scored tablets.

Mirtazapine (Remeron)

Mechanism of action: Presynaptic blocking of the alpha 2 adrenergic receptor. This results in the disinhibition of the NE and 5HT neurons, resulting in the increased release of NE and serotonin, enhancing activity of both systems in the brain. It also blocks 5HT2 and

5HT3 receptors, thereby improving tolerability. Finally, the antihistamine effect contributes to its sedation and weight-gaining properties.

Indications and uses: Adult patients with major depression, as well as depression associated with anxiety and panic.

Advantages: There are no gastrointestinal problems due to lack of 5HT3 stimulation. The sedation is helpful for insomniacs. It is also beneficial for those with anxiety, agitation, SSRI-induced sexual dysfunction, nausea, or stomach problems, as well as panic, weight loss, severe depression, and those who have lost their response to the SSRIs. There is a low likelihood of drug interactions, except for MAOIs. It may be added to SSRIs or venlafaxine to reduce the anxiety, nausea, and insomnia sometimes caused by these drugs.

Disadvantages: Sedation, dry mouth, weight gain, and the elevation of blood cholesterol levels. The gnawing hunger and increased appetite that can lead to overeating and weight gain can be helped by taking the over-the-counter medication Zantac, 75 to 150 mg, twice a day. This drug selectively blocks H2 receptors in the gut to decrease acid production and also improves movement of acid out of the esophagus and stomach.

Drug interactions: The drug interaction between Remeron and Valium is impairment of cognitive and motor skills. The effect is addictive when both drugs are taken simultaneously. Remeron should not be used in combination with an MAOI or within 14 days of initiating or discontinuing therapy with an MAOI.

Administration and dosage: The initial dose is 15 or 30 mg at bedtime. Lower doses are even more sedating than higher doses, which override the low-dose antihistamine effects (sedation is inversely related to dose).

Availability: 15- and 30-mg film-coated tablets.

Bupropion (Wellbutrin, Zyban)

Mechanism of action: Norepinephrine and dopamine reuptake inhibitor.

Indications and uses: Adult patients with major depression, those who don't tolerate the SSRIs, adult and childhood attention deficit disorder (ADD), and smoking cessation. It may also be useful for treating stimulant (amphetamine) withdrawal and craving. It has also been shown effective for bipolar disorder, particularly if the patient is cycling rapidly between manic and depressive states.

Advantages: Unique from all other antidepressants in that there is no effect on serotonin. Can be used in combination with SSRIs. There are minimal effects on sexual function. There are minimal cardio-vascular side effects compared to TCAs. Buproprion is especially good for patients with cognitive slowing, who are overweight, and who oversleep.

Disadvantages: Possibility of seizures with immediate release form of drug (only use sustained release SR form). Possibility of headache, nausea, agitation, insomnia, dry mouth, and constipation.

Notable contraindications: Wellbutrin is not to be used in anyone with a known seizure disorder or those with a history of bulimia or anorexia nervosa (due to the increased seizure risk).

Administration and dosage: The starting dose is 75- or 150-mg tablets, one to two times per day. The maximum dose is 450 mg in divided doses.

Buspirone (Buspar)

(**Note:** This drug is generally listed under antianxiety drugs because it has no indication for treatment of depression. It is being reviewed here because it is sometimes used in combination therapy in the treatment difficult cases of depression and anxiety, and because studies show that it does improve mood better than a placebo after three to four weeks.)

Mechanism of action: Selectively binds to the presynaptic 5HT1A autoreceptor, mimicking serotonin and resulting in decreased serotonin synthesis. Selectively binds to postsynaptic 5HT1A receptors, helping to normalize serotonin levels.

Indications and uses: Generalized anxiety disorder (GAD).

Advantages: It is nonaddictive and nonsedating compared to standard antianxiety drugs. There is no withdrawal syndrome upon discontinuation, maintains normal memory function, and there are very few incidents of sexual dysfunction.

Disadvantages and drug interactions: Combining with an MAOI may cause increased blood pressure. Progressive relief takes two to four weeks to achieve compared to more immediate effects of benzodiazepines for anxiety and panic attacks.

Dosage and administration: Start at 7.5 mg twice a day for the first week, then increase to 15 mg twice a day. Antidepressant combinations and augmentation strategies for difficult cases.

The serotonin strategies

When a patient has an unsatisfactory treatment response, a secondary agent may often be necessary to add to the first antidepressant. It is not uncommon for two or more drugs to be combined, especially in patients who have already found no success with a one-drug regimen. The psychopharmacologist will look for a combination of drugs in which one will cancel or at least mitigate the side effects of the other. Several strategies may be considered in view of the patient's diagnosis, history of response, and history of adverse reactions to medication.

In his book *Psychopharmacology of Antidepressants*, Stephen M. Stahl explains these more "heroic" strategies. By reviewing a few of them, we can understand the rationale a psychopharmacologist may use in treating these more difficult cases. The theory is that the depression will improve by increasing or potentiating the serotonin effect by adding a second drug with a different mechanism of serotonin enhancement to an SSRI. The three strategies are as follows:

❑ **Strategy 1.** Add 5HT1A receptor blocking drug buspirone (Buspar) to the SSRI. This will slow down the neuronal flow of serotonin and will cause the 5HT1A autoreceptor to downregulate, making more serotonin available in the synapse for the SSRI.

❑ **Strategy 2.** Add trazodone (Desyrel) or nefazadone (Serzone) to the SSRI. These drugs block the 5HT2 receptor and have some serotonin reuptake inhibition as well, again making more serotonin available for the SSRI to work better.

❑ **Strategy 3.** Add estrogen supplementation if the patient is estrogen deficient. It has been shown that female rats are not able to downregulate their 5HT2 receptors if their ovaries are removed. If estrogen is then given to these rats, they regain the ability to downregulate these receptors, improving synaptic serotonin levels and making the SSRIs more effective. This should be considered in peri- and postmenopausal women who do not respond adequately to antidepressants.

The noradrenergic strategies

To improve effectiveness of treatment targeted at augmenting the NE neurotransmitter system, a selective NRI like reboxetine or desipramine may be combined with:

❑ Bupropion (Wellbutrin), which is known to block both NE and dopamine reuptake.

❑ Bromocriptine, a dopamine enhancer.

❑ Pemoline, methylphenidate, and amphetamine, which are dopamine releasers.

Combining serotonin and noradrenegic strategies

Augmentation of both the 5HT and NE systems at the same time can be a powerful option if the patient's depression has not responded to other medical regimens. Those drugs that boost both the 5HT and NE systems as a single agent include the TCA clomipramine (Anafranil), and the atypical antidepressants mirtazapine (Remeron) and venlafaxine (Effexor). Venlafaxine in the morning complemented by mirtazapine at bedtime has been studied and shown to be an effective and safe combination. Both mirtazapine and venlafaxine can also be combined with either bupropion (Wellbutrin) or an SSRI. Nefazadone (Serzone) has also been used in combination with bupropion. Mixing TCAs with SSRIs and MAOIs with TCAs must be done with caution and careful monitoring.

Antidepressant augmentation strategies

Finally, it is not uncommon initially to add in a benzodiazapine antianxiety drug while waiting for an antidepressant to take effect. Many bipolar cases require an antidepressant with a mood stabilizer, such as lithium. Those with paranoid ideation or other psychotic features in bipolar disorders may also benefit from some of the newer antipsychotics, such as Zyprexa. Beta blockers are specifically helpful in cases of specific and social phobia where a predictable overactivation of the adrenergic autonomic system causes symptoms of palpitations, nausea, tremor, sweats, dizziness, and so forth, which can be blocked before they occur by a low dose of propanolol. Pindolol is also a beta blocker, but its action is directly in the synapse, where it helps to control serotonin levels. Thyroid supplements seem to improve the effectiveness of antidepressants as well, perhaps by their effect on the NE system, and the female cycle may occasionally need manipulation to help with the mood changes caused by dysregulation, or loss of the female hormones.

Anxiolytics

Benzodiazepines and buspirone are the primary drugs used to treat generalized anxiety disorders. No doubt more and more of the antidepressant drugs will be approved for generalized anxiety as time goes on, as we have already seen with venlafaxine (Effexor).

Benzodiazepines are commonly used at the outset of diagnosis because they are almost immediately effective. The rate of absorption of these drugs determines how quickly they will act, and how long they last depends on whether or not they are broken down in the body to secondary components that are still chemically active (active metabolites).

Buspirone (Buspar), already described above, is listed as an anxiolytic, or anti-anxiety, drug in the *Physician's Desk Reference* (*PDR*). It is the only marketed antianxiety drug that is not a tranquilizer. There is a one- to three-week delay before the onset of action, and the patient must be made aware of this lag time at the beginning of treatment. Although it does not have an indication for depression, there is considerable evidence that it possesses intrinsic antidepressant activity. Benefits for improving anxiety, especially in combination therapy, is well established. Unlike the benzodiazepines, buspirone is not addictive and has an excellent safety profile. Unlike lithium, it does not need to be monitored with laboratory tests.

Benzodiazepines also complement treatment with antidepressants, by counteracting the symptoms of agitation, anxiety, and insomnia that commonly accompany depression. They work by targeting the gamma-aminobutyric acid (GABA) neuronal system, the brain's major inhibitory transmitter system. Because antidepressant medication may take several weeks to improve the symptoms of anxiety and panic, it is very helpful to give the patient short-term control of these symptoms with the benzodiazepine drugs. Panic disorder usually requires the use of high-potency benzodiazepines, such as clonazepam (Klonopin) and alprazolam (Xanax). Medical treatment of panic disorder should also include an antidepressant approved for this indication.

Acute panic attacks may be treated in several ways, including a dose of 1 mg of lorazepam (Ativan) or alprazolam (Xanax) under the tongue in urgent cases. The longer-acting benzodiazepines, such as Klonopin, are used as mood stabilizers, ongoing generalized anxiety, and to help in the treatment of alcohol withdrawal. The shorter-acting drugs in this class, such as quazepam (Doral) and triazolam (Halcion) are used as sedatives for sleep and medical procedures such as endoscopy.

There are several side effects and problems with benzodiazepine drugs that must be considered. If the dose exceeds what's needed for sedation, slurred speech, balance problems, confusion, amnesia, errors in judgement, and increased anxiety and agitation can result. "Accidental deaths" have been caused by mixing these drugs with alcohol. Overdoses, as are often seen in suicide attempts, lead to respiratory depression, drop in blood pressure, coma, and death. Fortunately, there is now an antidote called flumanzenil that reverses the effects of benzodiazepines. It can be used by the emergency room physician in cases of overdose.

Abruptly stopping sedative drugs after regular use can cause serious and even fatal seizures. More mild symptoms associated with sedative withdrawal include disturbed sleep, depression, irritability, anxiety, poor concentration, tremor, nausea, and muscle aches. Withdrawal effects are more severe with the shorter-acting benzodiazepines. There are no significant side effects on any systems other than the brain.

Other sedative and hypnotic drugs used in sleep and anxiety disorders include phenobarbital, chloral hydrate (Noctec), hydroxizine (Vistaril), and zolpidem (Ambien).

Thyroid hormone supplementation

It has long been observed that patients with abnormally high or low levels of thyroid hormone are vulnerable to psychological disturbances.

If the body produces too many thyroid hormones, a patient may become agitated, tremulous, and anxious. Too little of these hormones may cause depression, lethargy, and hypersomnolence.

In the early 1970s, several studies showed the value of thyroid hormones, especially T3, in augmenting the effectiveness of tricyclic antidepressants (TCAs) and in speeding up their onset of action. This seemed particularly true in depressed women. Later studies showed the use of T4 as a helpful drug in augmenting mood stabilizers in the treatment of bipolar disorder, especially for the rapid cycling subtype. The mechanism of action of T3 augmentation is likely due to the important interactions of T3 with the various neurotransmitters, particularly norepinephrine. A common augmentation strategy is to use Cytomel (T3), 5 mg daily.

Female hormone supplementation

The mood swings accompanying the menstrual period and the perimenopausal and postmenopausal times of life are well documented, as are the beneficial effects of hormonal replacement therapy on improving the effectiveness of medical treatment for depression and anxiety in women with hormonal instability.

Younger women may benefit from a birth-control pill if periods are erratic and cause significant mood changes associated with premenstrual syndrome (PMS). The perimenopausal woman, who may be skipping periods or having them closer together, can be started on an androgen supplement in the form of a progesterone cream, and then started on estrogen replacement with the cessation of menstrual periods.

Hormonal manipulation and replacement therapy offers many options, including combination pills taken once a day (such as premarin/provera, Prempro, estrogen/testosterone, Estratest), patches used once or twice a week (such as Climara, Vivelle, Estroderm), cycling birth-control pills, or injections every three months (Deprovera). The variety of options make an endocrine or gynecological evaluation helpful when hormonal treatment may be indicated.

Mood stabilizers

Mood stabilizers are used primarily to stop the cycling between manic and depressive states in patients with bipolar illness. Drugs with a wide variety of mechanisms of action have been found to be useful for this purpose, including benzodiazepines, anticonvulsants, neuroleptics (antipsychotics), lithium, calcium channel blockers, and even narcotics. The primary drugs for this purpose are listed below.

Lithium

In approximately 70 percent of patients with bipolar illness, lithium significantly decreases the frequency of both manic and depressive episodes and is used as a prophylactic (preventative) drug. Patients who cycle rapidly back and forth between manic and depressive attacks (at least four cycles per year) usually do not respond well to preventative lithium therapy. Some continue to improve with long-term therapy. The effective dose range for acute mania is 1,200 to 1,800 mg per day, but the dose is usually half this when given to augment an antidepressant drug for long-term prevention.

Lithium can be taken all at once, once a day, or in divided doses with food to prevent nausea. Monitoring of lithium blood levels may be indicated every one to 12 months, depending on the individual and length of treatment.

Many side effects are possible, including nausea, fine tremors (which can be treated with propanolol), slight muscle weakness, and sleepiness. Many of these are transient and go away with continued use. Endocrine changes such as a decrease in thyroid function and a particular type of diabetes may occur during treatment, but resolve within eight weeks of discontinuation of therapy.

Lithium in combination with benzodiazepines causes sexual dysfunction in about 50 percent of men, may exacerbate asthma, and may worsen certain cases of psoriasis. Long-term use may have adverse effects on the kidneys in some individuals and may also affect memory and emotional reactivity. Toxicity usually occurs at levels above two meq/L (meq/L = miliequivalents per liter). Care must be used if lithium is used with certain diuretics or ACE inhibitors, as these drugs may increase blood lithium to toxic levels.

Benzodiazepines

Klonopin at bedtime, in doses ranging from 1-4 mg, or 1-2 mg every four to six hours, is helpful in controlling the acute behavioral symptoms of mania, and is a good alternative to the neuroleptic drugs because of fewer side effects. Doses up to 16 mg per day are sometimes necessary.

Neuroleptics

Once only used in cases of psychosis such as schizophrenia, neuroleptic drugs are now used for augmentation and improved clinical response in a number of psychological illnesses. In bipolar disorder, haloperidol (Haldol) is used for acute manic symptoms of agitation and psychosis. The dose in the hospital setting is five to 10 mg orally or by injection every two to three hours until the symptoms calm down. After this initial use, the drug is decreased as another mood stabilizer is added for more long-term use (usually lithium). Newer neuroleptics, such as Zyprexa, have fewer side effects and may be used more frequently in the future.

Anticonvulsants

The anticonvulsants represent a diverse group of agents. Originally developed to control seizures, they have also been found useful for their effects on mood. Valproic acid and carbamazepine have been shown to work as mood stabilizers and antidepressants, although they are rarely used in this latter role due to side effects. Recently, the anticonvulsants lamotrigine and gabapentin have been reported to produce anti manic and antidepressant activity, but they require further study.

Valproic acid

This antiseizure drug's activity is at least partially due to its effects on the GABA neurotransmitter system. It is sometimes used in preference to lithium as first-line treatment for mania because of its better safety profile. Valproic acid has also been shown to improve the course of panic disorder and migraine headaches. Treatment is usually started at 250 mg, three times a day, and may be increased to achieve therapeutic levels in the bloodstream. Liver tests and blood counts, as well as drug blood levels, need to be monitored.

Carbamazepine

This anticonvulsant stabilizes the activity of cell membranes and is used to treat bipolar patients who have rapid cycling between mania and depression or patients who cannot tolerate lithium. It is usually effective at doses of 800 to 1,600 mg per day. It has also been used with success in resistant depression, alcohol withdrawal, panic disorder, and patients who have difficulty controlling their behavior.

It has also been used in patients who have previously abused stimulants (such as amphetamines), especially in patients who have posttraumatic stress disorder with poor impulse control. Several drugs increase blood levels of carbamazepine and should be used with caution. Blood counts and liver function tests should be monitored as well.

Lamotrigine and gabapentin

Both of these newer anticonvulsants have an indication for use in seizures, but they are also showing promise for use in augmentation therapy of depression and bipolar disorder, especially for rapid cycling (four or more mood shifts per year). Lamotrigine provokes the release of the excitatory amino acids glutamate and aspartate, and therein may lie its mechanism of action.

Side effects are usually mild and may include headache, dizziness, double vision, and nausea. A rash occurs in 10 percent of patients and is an indication to stop the drug. Dosing starts at 25 to 50 mg per day and may be increased slowly. Gabapentin is structurally related to GABA, but it has not been shown to interact with GABA or GABA receptors. Its mechanism of action is unknown. There are reports suggesting its possible role as an adjunct in the treatment of refractory bipolar illness. The effective dose is 900 to 1,800 mg per day in three divided doses. The most common side effects are fatigue, drowsiness, and dizziness.

Beta blockers
Propanolol (Inderal) and atenolol (Tenormin)

Propanolol has been around a long time and has been given a variety of odd jobs in the garden of health care due to its capacity to block beta adrenergic receptors and thereby block the effects of excess adrenaline and adrenergic stimulation. It is very effective in preventing certain forms of migraine headaches and prevents the racing heart and palpitations seen in mitral valve prolapse. Those with social phobia have found that it blocks some of the more bothersome symptoms, such as fast heart rate and tremors, caused by autonomic arousal that they experience when forced to face their dysfunction, such as giving a talk in front of a group of peers.

Atenolol is a longer-acting beta blocker often used in the patient with hyperarousal and anxiety in the setting of concurrent high blood pressure. These drugs are not used as primary agents in the treatment of panic disorder because they do not block panic and do not lessen the cognitive and emotional experience of fear. They may, however, be used as an adjunct to other therapies to reduce some of the physical symptoms that occur with autonomic stimulation.

Pindolol

Even though beta blockers are often cited as a cause of depression, this particular one is on the list of drugs used to treat depression. It especially seems useful in enhancing the actions of the SSRIs by helping to regulate serotonin levels between nerve cells. Those with severe asthma or allergies may experience a worsening of these conditions while on pindolol.

Calcium channel blockers

These drugs, which block the movement of calcium across the ion channels of the cell membrane, (for example, verapamil [Calan]), have been used in bipolar states that have failed to respond to lithium, caramazepine, or valproic acid. It has also been found in preliminary reports to be helpful in panic disorder. A closer look into these drugs, which are typically used for high blood pressure and angina, was indicated when it was realized that a number of psychoactive drugs have calcium channel-blocking properties, including lithium, antidepressants, neuroleptics, and carbamazepine. Although safer than lithium or carbamazepine during pregnancy, verapamil must be stopped before delivery because it can cause a decrease in the uterine contractility.

Other medical and surgical treatments

Electroconvulsive therapy (ECT)

Electroconvulsive therapy is the most effective treatment for severe depression that responds poorly to other techniques. Approximately 70 to 85 percent of patients with severe depression respond favorably to ECT, especially those with agitation and delusions. It is also effective in manic disorders and psychoses during pregnancy, when the use of drugs may be contraindicated. Comparative studies have proven that ECT is more effective than medical treatments in patients with severe depression.

Many people resist getting this form of treatment, even after several physicians have advised them that they should benefit greatly by getting it. In *Undercurrents*, Martha Manning chronicles her own depression and experience with ECT, and comments on the day she found the address of a gun shop: "I didn't want to die because I hated myself—I wanted to die because I loved myself enough to want this pain to end. However, I listened to my daughter singing in the shower and knew that if I killed myself I would stop that song. The next day, I checked myself in for ECT."

The procedure is performed in the hospital setting under a short-acting general anesthesia and a muscle relaxant to prevent physical spasm, with the goal being to apply a high enough electrical current to the brain to induce a generalized central nervous system seizure (body convulsions are not needed). The patient is connected to the heart monitor and electroencephalogram before treatment is initiated. Once the patient is unconscious, an electric stimulus lasting a few seconds is applied via electrodes attached to the temples. This causes a seizure in the brain that usually lasts about 50 seconds, long enough to stimulate a change in brain chemistry but not long enough to cause any problems.

Seizures can be induced by electrical or chemical means, but electricity is more reliable and simple. When a seizure occurs, the brain responds at the cellular level by regulating neurotransmitter and receptor interactions. By this mechanism, the healthy benefits are thought to arise. The patient wakes up in approximately 10 minutes in the recovery room, eats a meal, and is then taken to his or her room.

Serious complications are rare, occurring in less than one in 1,000 cases. Some memory loss and confusion may follow ECT, as one would expect after a seizure. The degree of disturbance correlates to the number and frequency of treatments.

Poor patient understanding of the technique of ECT and lack of acceptance are the biggest obstacles to the use of this valuable technique. It's unfortunate that more people don't hear the success stories of ECT. Manning writes further about the effectiveness of her own ECT treatment: "Before, I was aware of every swallow of water, that each was just too much work. Afterward, I thought, 'Do regular people feel this way all the time?' It's like you've been not in on a great joke for the whole of your life."

RTMS

Repeated transcranial magnetic stimulation (RTMS) is a next-generation device being developed by Robert Post at the National Institute for Mental Health. The idea is to use fluxes in magnetic fields to stimulate the brain, without producing seizures. In the past, electric stimulation that fell short of producing seizures was not effective in improving symptoms. Magnetic fluxes travel easily through the skull, unlike electric currents. If this treatment does prove effective in the treatment of depression, it will not have the side effects of memory loss and disorientation seen with ECT.

Phototherapy

Light therapy hardly sounds like medical intervention, but it belongs here as a scientifically studied and physician-prescribed remedy. This modality is used to treat the depression of seasonal affective disorder (SAD) and consists of exposure (at a distance of three feet) to a light source of 2,500 lux for two hours daily. Light exposures may work through effects on the pineal gland and alteration of biorhythm through melatonin mechanisms. Light visors are also available for greater mobility and an adjustable light intensity. Some patients may do better on a morning and night exposure regimen.

Surgical options for refractory cases

If all else fails, surgery may be an option to consider. However, when people think about psychosurgery, it is difficult not to conjure up images of *One Flew Over the Cuckoo's Nest* and the protagonist's final taming by way of a lobotomy. This procedure involved the severing of the prefrontal lobes in patients with severe neuropsychiatric disorders. It was performed approximately 5,000 times a year in the United States in the late 1940s and early 50s, with up to one in 15 patients dying from complications of the procedure.

This procedure, fortunately, is a far cry from the cingulotomy procedure used today. In this operation, the scalp is frozen locally and the neurosurgeon drills a small hole in the front of the skull. Through this small opening, an electrode is introduced into a specific area of brain tissue and a current is applied to destroy an area measuring approximately eight by 18 millimeters.

Up to 70 percent of patients who undergo this procedure have some degree of improvement, and about 30 percent are significantly better. This track record is remarkable, considering these are the patients with the most severe cases — those that have not responded to all other forms of therapy.

Removing this small area creates a trauma to which the brain must respond to. The delayed and indirect effect on other parts of the brain causes a gradual change for the better over the weeks and months following the procedure. Massachusetts General Hospital is the leading center in the United States for this surgery, performing only 15 to 20 cases per year due to a difficult protocol that one must pass before being approved for the operation.

Summing up for now

You have every reason to feel a bit dizzy at the range and complication of treatment options available for anxiety, panic, and depression. So as not to overload this already full chapter, we will reserve a discussion of other common treatment options for later chapters. The information presented here, however, should underline the importance of working with a trusted health professional—someone who knows you well and knows available treatment options. The terms and concepts of this chapter should also give you insight into your treatment. A physician's prescription will no longer be a "mystery pill" for you. At least, in a general way, you will understand what that medication is attempting to do within your body. You will be better prepared to observe specific improvements in your symptoms and to record possible side effects of medication. In a word, you will *participate* in your treatment.

Barbara...A.P.D. and visits to the doctor

In my case, A.P.D. symptoms first began to seriously interrupt big parts of my life (vacations, social interaction, sports participation, work responsibilities, and so forth) more than two decades ago. I'm feeling a mixture of embarrassment and guilt to admit that it's been going on that long. If I were an alcoholic, I think I would feel the same sense of shame at not being better able to get control of such a destructive intruder into my life.

In those years (the early 1970s) many general practitioners didn't know quite what to say to people like me who came in with the bizarre range of symptoms associated with A.P.D. Here's a typical script from my twenty or so visits to doctors in those years. (Why didn't I go straight to a psychiatrist? I didn't have any better idea of what I was experiencing than my general practitioner did. And "shrinks" in those years were something you laughed at with Rowan and Martin on "Laugh-In." I wasn't crazy. Something was physically wrong.)

Visit 1: "Doctor, my pulse gets very rapid and sometimes irregular when I have to get up in front of people at work or at church."
Reply: (after tests) "Barbara, there's nothing physically wrong with your heart. I think you're just experiencing stress. It's all in your head."

Visit 5: "Doctor, I'm still getting feelings like I can't breathe and that my insides are just going wild. It isn't just making presentations at work—It's flying on airplanes, crossing bridges when I'm driving, and even on the subway coming to your office today."
Reply: (after thyroid, hypoglycemia, among other tests): "Barbara, all your tests are absolutely normal. You're the model of health. A lot of my patients would love to have your basic blood chemistry and good blood pressure. But we can put you into a clinic for a full workup if you want."

Visit 10: ($2,000 later): "Doctor, this is getting really bad. I'm having these feelings of terrible anxiety almost every time I leave the house. Can't we find out what's wrong with me?"
Reply: (after EEG, epilepsy workup, and additional tests): "Barbara, we still haven't been able to diagnose what's going on with any precision. It may be just psychosomatic. But just knowing that it's all in your head will probably come as a big relief to you."

This scenario, of course, is hard on the well-intentioned family doctor of the 1970s. Perhaps a referral would have been made earlier to a psychologist or psychiatrist (although similarly unproductive scripts could be written of those kind of trips as well!). Valium or its equivalent probably would have been prescribed along the way, with the usual result of temporary relief, then rebound anxiety, increasing drug reliance, the physician's unwillingness to increase dosages and authorize refills...followed by the patient's defection to begin with another physician, and a year later, another physician, and so forth.

Here's my point: I have spent a small fortune trying to find something devastatingly wrong with my heart, brain, lungs, blood, liver, kidneys, pancreas, and everything in between. People like me with A.P.D. desperately want to put a title, a name, a socially recognized label on their physical symptoms in order to externalize the beast and treat it like any other physical ill.

In my worst moments, I have almost wanted to be diagnosed with cancer or some progressive heart disease so that I could announce to my relatives, "I'd love to attend the family reunion at Yellowstone Park next summer, but unfortunately I have cancer and have to conserve my energy." Or to tell my boss, "I would be glad to fly to Cleveland to make that big presentation, but my physician won't let me fly due to my heart condition." Or to tell my husband, "I would do anything for you and the kids—anything—but I'm stuck with this darn brain tumor."

None of that works with A.P.D. symptoms, of course. I can't tell relatives, "Can't make it to Yellowstone, Bro and Sis, because I'm scared to travel and I feel like I'm going to freak out when I'm far from home and help." And I can't tell my boss the real reason why I've evaded so many business trips—so I make up one more lame excuse about a death in the extended family or a sudden illness for one of the kids. Saddest of all, I can't fully explain to my husband and certainly not to my kids that Mom struggles day by day and hour by hour with fears and feelings she can't exactly name or describe.

Since my early visits to my family doctor in the 1970s, a name has been put on my symptoms. Most magazines by this time have published several articles for the general public on anxiety, panic, and depression. Famous writers (Art Buchwald, William Styron, among others) have written eloquently about their struggles with depression. Finally, there is a label out there that presents A.P.D. distress as a bona fide illness, treatable in all the various ways presented in this book.

But for me, and I suspect thousands of other A.P.D. sufferers, this new label still carries with it the threat of social stigma or at least social suspicion. "Barbara can't go to Cleveland because she has an anxiety disorder," I imagine my boss saying to my colleagues at work, "and Jill can't go because she's in the last month of pregnancy." I leave it to you: Which of these two explanations will continue to raise eyebrows and ruin reputations?

8 | What About Herbs, Vitamins, and Supplements?

According to the World Health Organization, approximately 80 percent the world's population relies on herbs for health care needs. In many developed countries, including Japan, Germany, France, Italy, and Australia, herbs are commonly prescribed in medical practice. Although herbs are popular in America ($4 billion spent in 1998), that use does not begin to compare per capita to the $7.5 billion Germans spent in the same year for herbs.

The number of Americans turning to alternative medicine practitioners and herbal remedies is growing for several reasons. Some people believe conventional physicians write prescriptions in an unthinking, reflexive manner without regard for the overall health of the patient, and that natural medicines are better and safer for the body. A 1997 national survey conducted by *Prevention* magazine reported that approximately 32 percent of adult Americans frequently use herbal medicines.

People are also afraid of the drugs used in conventional medicine. They may have read or heard that more than 150,000 deaths in the United States each year are attributed to both prescription and over-the-counter drugs. Of course, they do not stop to consider the lives saved and improved by modern pharmaceuticals. The fact is that at least half the time, patients failed to follow the directions on how to take the medication given by the doctor. Patients also frequently mix their medications with alcohol or other drugs not approved by their physician.

Other people balk at the cost of modern drugs. Herbal alternatives may be an appealingly affordable option, especially for those without prescription benefits as part of their health insurance. Because consumers in the United States are spending billions of dollars annually for alternative care, the medical profession is taking heed of this demand for more options in the healing process. Large university hospitals are starting to spawn "complementary" medicine programs that make herbal medications available to those patients who prefer this option. Many medical schools have added complementary medicine courses for those physicians who are interested in offering herbal medicines and natural healing programs in their future medical practices. Even insurance companies and some HMOs are beginning to offer coverage for alternative treatments, perhaps because of increased acceptance in the medical community, perhaps because they are cheaper.

With a track record for improving symptoms of anxiety, panic, and depression, there is much to be said for herbs. As a rule, these substances are milder and slower acting than many prescription alternatives. For these reasons, herbs may not be the first option for the "now" generation, unwilling to accept the longer course of time that herbal medications often take to exert their effects. These patients (of all ages) want the strongest thing available. They will not return in the future if offered an herb instead of a prescription.

People suffering from stress will often turn to short-term, addictive drugs, such as alcohol, cigarettes, muscle relaxants, sleeping pills, tranquilizers or recreational drugs for temporary relief. This only gives them a new problem to be stressed about. It is the job of all physicians and health professionals to encourage a patient to let his or her body heal itself whenever possible, and to be sure the patient is using all possible natural methods for healing before resorting to a drug.

That's where herbs play a valuable role. The following herbal medicines have been selected by Dr. Harold H. Bloomfield because of their potential usefulness in treating depression, anxiety, and the symptoms that these disorders may cause.

Herbal remedies

Kava kava

Coming from the root of the pepper tree (Piper methysticum), kava kava was traditionally consumed by Polynesian chieftains of the South Pacific Islands during ceremonial rites. Kava kava is said to have calming effects without the mental impairment or depressed mood sometimes caused by the benzodiazepine tranquilizers. The pills come in strengths of 100 to 250 mg and can be taken up to three times a day. Oversedation has occurred in patients who mixed kava kava with benzodiazepine tranquilizers. Taking this herb for more than 25 weeks is generally not recommended.

Many European health boards have approved kava kava for the treatment of anxiety and insomnia. Kava kava has been studied and found to be superior to placebo in improving the symptoms of anxiety, as well as being well tolerated with mild and rare adverse reactions. Anything can be overdone, and those abusing this herb have had more serious reactions including yellowing of the skin, liver test abnormalities, muscle spasms, and breathing difficulty. Taken as directed, and without mixing with alcohol or sedative drugs, kava kava is a helpful first-line treatment for mild anxiety disorders.

Hypericum (St. John's wort)

Hypericum perforatum, also known as St. John's wort (wort means "plant," not something on the bottom of Saint John's foot), is a perennial plant with bright yellow flowers that bloom annually around the time of St. John's birthday, June 20. It has been used for at least 2,500 years as a folk remedy for anxiety, worry, and sleeping problems. It was prescribed by Hippocrates for "nervous unrest."

Hypericum is substantially less expensive than prescription antidepressants and is available over the counter. The antianxiety effects are due to its antidepressant effects, which, like all modern antidepressants, take a few weeks to kick in. The herbal drug seems to work by enhancing the three key neurotransmitter systems (norepinephrine, dopamine, and serotonin), as well as increasing the activity of the GABA system, which has a tranquilizing effect on the central nervous system.

Because hypericum is an SSRI, it should not be taken with a MAO inhibitor because of the risk of dangerously high blood pressure, anxiety, fever, confusion, and muscle tension. One should stop any MAO inhibitor for four weeks before starting hypericum or any other antidepressant. Changing from a prescription antidepressant to hypericum should be done very slowly and under the guidance of a physician. This herb may be considered for mild to moderate depression that is not complicated by other diagnoses. It has a remarkable safety record over centuries of use. Multiple studies have shown it to have an effectiveness on a par with some modern antidepressants, with a safety profile and tolerability better than synthetic antidepressants.

This herb has a place in the medical arsenal of treatments for anxiety and depression, but the decision regarding which drug to initiate should be made only after a professional evaluation by a physician. Since the FDA does not permit manufacturers of St. John's wort to make claims about its use for treating depression, it is not packaged with patient information about the effective treatment of depression. That lack of information can be disastrous.

Patients with major depression need ongoing antidepressant medication for at least six to nine months, according to the Agency for Health Care Policy and Research (AHCPR). Even if you recover right away, the risk of relapse is high if medication is not continued for the prescribed course. Many patients taking St. John's wort have no guidance as to when they should expect to see benefits or how long they should take it. If you're sick enough to take the wort, you're sick enough to get the work up. A typical dosage is 300 mg of an extract standardized to .3 percent hypericin, once to three times daily. It is not known if food affects absorption, so it's probably a good idea to take it on an empty stomach.

Valerian

Otherwise known as "nature's Valium," valerian extract comes from the root stock of *Valerian officinalis*, which has been used for thousands of years in India and China as a sedative and sleep enhancer. It probably works like the benzodiazepines, such as Valium, by increasing the activity of GABA, the sedative-like neurotrans-mitter. Valerian has been found to be helpful in inducing sleep, reducing nightmares, and preventing early-morning awakening. Valerian is the most widely used sedative in Europe and its use is growing throughout the world. A 1996 study by Gerhart and Associates showed a five-fold increase in side effects with Valium compared to valerian. This research organization is best known for its studies of herbal remedies. In this double-blind, placebo-controlled study, researchers compared valerian to benzodiazepines and a placebo in the treatment of insomnia. Ten percent of the subjects treated with valerian complained of side effects, compared to 50 percent of the benzodiazepine group. Valerian and benzodiazepines were found to be similarly effective for the treatment of insomnia, but valerian caused less daytime drowsiness and did not seem to cause memory or concentration impairment at levels higher than the placebo.

Like all sedatives, it should not be combined with alcohol and it is not recommended to take valerian for more than six months. There are some reports of adverse effects, such as headaches, nervousness, restlessness, and palpitations, but these are rare.

Chamomile

Chamomile (*Matricaria recutita*) is widely used in the Western world for anxiety, nervous stomach, and relaxation. The active ingredient, apigenin, causes sedation by acting on the GABA receptors in the brain, just as benzodiazepines like Valium. A member of the daisy family, chamomile is harvested just before the flower heads bloom.

A few people may be allergic to chamomile, especially if they have a ragweed or chrysanthemum allergy, so be careful the first time you try it. Chamomile tea has only a small percentage of the sedative chemicals compared to the herb, but is still useful as a stomach calming agent and mild relaxant. The herb is available in a standardized extract containing 1.2 percent apigenin and 0.5 percent essential oils. Follow the directions on the bottle of extract to provide a dose sufficient for mild sedation when needed. The oil is often used in aromatherapy for stress relief.

California poppy

The California poppy (*Eschscholtzia californica*) has gained in popularity as a sleep aid and stress reducer. It gets its name from the Russian physician who discovered the plant, Doctor Eschscholtz. The California poppy is in the same family as the opium poppy (but not the same genus), from whence the narcotics codeine and morphine are derived. Its active chemicals, known as alkaloids, are less powerful and not addictive.

California poppy is sold in a tincture (a liquid extract), which should be mixed with your favorite juice to disguise the taste. Thirty drops is the usual dose, but follow the directions on the bottle as the strengths of extracts can vary.

Hops

Humulus lupulus, the hops plant, is a perennial vine. The hairs of its scaly, conelike fruits contain these medicinal substances. Used for hundreds of years in Europe to flavor and preserve beer, hops was known to have sedating properties. (The pickers who accidentally ingested them were sometimes found asleep on the job!) A sedative chemical known as dimethylvinyl has been identified as the active ingredient causing its tranquilizing properties. Hops loses up to 90 percent of its potency after nine months of storage, so it should be used as fresh as possible. It is available as a 5.2 percent extract or 2 percent essential oil and can be combined with valerian to improve sleep and enable the user to feel alert and rested the next day.

Passion flower

Passiflora incarnata, the passion flower, is native to North America and is used for nervousness, restlessness, anxiety, insomnia, and irritability. When taken as a sleeping aid, it has no hangover sedation in the morning. Passion flower is available in a standardized extract containing 3.5 to 4 percent of the active ingredient isovitexin (flavonoids); 200 to 300 mg of the extract can be taken one hour before bedtime.

Ginsengs

According to Dr. Harold H. Bloomfield, "Although you cannot avoid stress, an astounding group of herbal medicines, called *adaptogens*, can strengthen the body's ability to *adapt* to stress. Adaptogens, also called nerve tonics, help normalize the functions of the body and make it more resistant to stress." Adaptogens must fulfill the following three criteria: They must be innocuous, causing no harm over long-term use; increase resistance to stress; and improve physical and mental performance.

Adaptogenic herbs contain multiple constituents that are able to accomplish opposing results when isolated. For instance, one component may raise blood pressure, while another lowers it. Or one may increase blood sugar while another lowers it. The theory of how these drugs work involves the body's ability to utilize these various constituents of the herb in the amounts it needs to restore its own internal balance.

The most well-known adaptogens are the ginsengs. Some studies have indicated that these herbs have effects on blood oxygenation and blood sugar metabolism and may stimulate immune system and adrenal function. They are especially helpful to the individual who is physically overworked and burnt out.

Asian ginseng

Panax ginseng has been in use for more than 4,000 years and is a small perennial plant found in China, Korea, and Japan. The active drug is derived from the dried root and root hairs. High-quality wild ginseng is extremely hard to find and very expensive. Small studies seem to support the claims that Asian ginseng improves mental concentration, physical performance, general energy level, memory, alertness, and mood. It may also lower blood cholesterol and decrease the risk of heart attack through the action of an agent that prevents blood clots.

Because it is a stimulant that increases adrenal function, it is not recommended if your anxiety is not under control, or if you have bipolar disorder, heart palpitations, are pregnant, or have asthma. The usual dosage is 100 mg of 13 percent extract two times a day.

The dosage for ginseng powder is 1,500 mg daily in two separate doses. Some experts recommend a two weeks on/two weeks off dosing regimen.

American ginseng

Panax quinquefolius is considered less stimulating than Asian ginseng and is preferred by many Asians who find their own ginseng too strong. It takes five years of cultivation to produce a mature root. Most American ginseng is produced in Wisconsin and British Columbia. The wild plant is endangered because of the extensive hunting and harvesting of the plant in nature. Collection and sale of the native plant requires a permit and is therefore very expensive.

Native American Indians used American ginseng to strengthen mental powers and to treat nausea and vomiting. The American frontiersman, Daniel Boone, helped export American ginseng, and the wealthy and politically connected Astor family of Maidenhead, England, made its fortune by shipping it to China. The usual dosage is 100 mg of 13 percent extract taken twice a day.

Siberian ginseng

Siberian ginseng, *Eleutherococcus senticosus* (also known as eleuthero), is not a species of *Panax* and is therefore not a traditional ginseng. It does have similar adaptogen characteristics. Its active chemicals, called eleutherosides, are located similarly in the root structures. The benefits that have been reported include helping adaptation to climactic extremes of heat, cold, and altitude, while improving hearing and visual activity. It has been advertised as a low-cost substitute for *Panax* ginseng. Those with mild anxiety and insomnia should consider eleuthero over *Panax* species ginseng.

Studies of patients with general anxiety, irritability, and extreme exhaustion showed significant improvement in subjective sense of well-being. Germany's Commission E health authorities have allowed Siberian ginseng to be labeled as a tonic against stress, for fortification in times of fatigue, debility, and convalescence (as well as in times of decreased work capacity and poor mental concentration). The usual dose is 0.5 to 6.0 mL of a 33 percent extract, taken one to three times daily. The other form available is a .8 percent eleutheroside extract and the dose range is 180 to 360 mg per day in divided doses. The Sunsource company has made a new supplement called "Harmonex," which combines Siberian ginseng and St. John's wort extract to help maintain physical and emotional balance.

Milk thistle

Milk thistle is another adaptogen widely used to enhance liver function in hopes of improving the liver's ability to detoxify harmful chemicals in the internal environment. The herb is thought to prevent and reverse liver damage caused by alcohol, as well as environmental pollutants, chemical pesticides, auto exhaust, and other byproducts. Few physicians would argue with the idea of doing something healthful for your liver! Approximately 78 percent of adult Americans have some level of chronic liver damage, according to studies published by the *Journal of the American Medical Association*. Nearly 2,000 years ago it was being recommended by the Greek physician Dioscorides for the purpose of treating liver damage from toxic poisoning.

This thistle-topped weed has a prickly purple flower with seeds that contain antioxidant flavonoids. One of these chemicals, silymarin, has been demonstrated in medical research to protect liver cells from damage caused by harmful free radicals produced by stress and toxic chemicals and to stimulate regeneration when these cells do sustain damage. It is thought to be especially valuable in liver damage caused by alcohol. A 200 mg pill of milk thistle extract contains 80 percent (or 160 mg) of silymarin, which should be taken three times a day.

Ginkgo biloba

If it is true, as stated by Dr. Ashley Montagu, that "the goal of life is to die young — as late as possible," then those suffering from anxiety about getting old and senile will be relieved to hear about some of the benefits that many experience from the herb ginkgo. Ginkgo sales in Germany alone in 1996 topped $163 million and more than 120,000 physicians worldwide write more than 10 million prescriptions for it each year, accounting for $500 million in sales.

It is made from the ginkgo tree, the oldest living tree species in the world, which has survived basically unchanged for over three hundred million years in China. It was observed to be the only plant to survive the atomic blast at Hiroshima. It seems to be remarkably resistant to disease, insects, pollution, and radiation. Individual trees can live more than a thousand years. The October 1997 issue of the *Journal of the American Medical Association* presented research showing that ginkgo biloba extract appears to slow Alzheimer's disease. The study, performed by Dr. Pierre LeBars at the New York Institute for Medical Research, found that 27 percent of those who took 120 mg of the herb daily for six months or longer improved their mental abilities in the areas of memory, reasoning, and ability to learn, compared to 14 percent of those in the placebo group. Some German studies have found a higher dose of 240 mg to be more effective. Many studies on tens of thousands of patients attest to the effectiveness of ginkgo in improving the problems associated with poor blood flow in the elderly, especially in the brain.

In the United States, the extract is sold under the trade names Ginkgold and Ginkgo-D. The active ingredient, called Egb761, has demonstrated both antianxiety and antidepressant activities. Egb761 has been shown to globally increase brain neurotransmitter function by inhibiting the reuptake of serotonin, norepinephrine, dopamine, and acetylcholine. It is also thought to improve oxygen and glucose utilization while increasing blood flow and delivery of oxygen and nutrients to the tissues. Ginkgo has been recommended by herbalists for the treatment of many of the presumed symptoms of aging, including anxiety and depression, memory loss, poor concentration, diminished intellectual capacity, and other ailments that have to do with poor circulation, such as macular degeneration, poor circulation in the legs, impotence due to diminished penile blood flow, diabetic tissue damage, Raynaud's phenomenon, and some headache-based disorders.

Because of the blood-thinning effects caused by its ability to prevent platelets in the blood from forming clots, ginkgo biloba use should be brought to the attention of your doctor if you are taking a blood thinner or if you are being considered for any surgical procedure. To date, at least four reports of spontaneous bleeding in association with use of ginkgo biloba have been published. One involved a 70-year-old man who started bleeding inside the eye one week after starting the herb at a dosage of 40 mg twice a day. Another was a 33-year-old woman who developed bleeding inside the brain after taking ginkgo at 60 mg twice a day for almost two years. Until further information is available, patients who are taking garlic, vitamin E, warfarin (coumadin), aspirin, or other platelet-inhibiting drugs should use ginkgo with caution and the advice of your physician.

Reishi, a medicinal mushroom

For thousands of years, Taoist monks have used reishi mushrooms (*Ganoderma lucidum*) to promote inner calmness and deepen their meditative powers, as well as improve health and longevity. Living a long life has always been a strong cultural value for the Chinese. These mushrooms are becoming more popular in the U.S. for reducing anxiety and insomnia. In ancient times, they were used for asthma, bronchitis, liver disease, and high blood pressure. Triterpene acids, one of the active ingredients in reishi, has been shown to effectively lower blood pressure. The mushrooms also contain certain polysaccharides that have antibacterial and anti-inflammatory properties. Reishi extract is standardized with 4 percent triterpenes and 10 percent polysaccharides. The usual dose is 250 to 350 mg, taken three times daily.

Traditional Chinese medicine

Traditional Chinese medicine (TCM) is one of the oldest written medical systems, using herbs in conjunction with a dualistic Taoist philosophy of yin and yang. Yin (the cool, dim, yielding, and feminine component) and yang (the warm, bright, dominant, and masculine component) are viewed as the two opposing forces in all living things. In order to enjoy good health and physical and emotional harmony, every human being in the TCM perspective must maintain a balance of yin and yang. Stress and anxiety can lead to a depletion of the yin component, which can be restored with a combination of herbs, dietary adjustments, qigong exercises (exercises that incorporate deep breathing, stretching, and balancing in gentle, controlled, and flowing movements), massage, and acupuncture.

As explained by Gary Kaplan, DO (Doctor of Osteopathy), who consulted on an article on acupuncture in the June 15, 1999, issue of *Patient Care* magazine:

> The intent of Chinese medicine is the same as that of Western medicine: to restore homeostasis of the body and mind. The Chinese are more interested in who a person is in totality, in how someone ended up in his present state. They look for patterns of disharmony. In addition to asking the standard questions about major illnesses and presenting complaints, a practitioner might also ask about food cravings, the patient's vacation preferences, his relationship with his parents, and the like. The information may not make sense in Western medicine, which focuses on specific symptoms of the presenting condition. A physician who is not trained in the Chinese way would not know what to do with these findings.

Many combinations of herbs used in TCM are designed to maintain the proper balance to promote health (that is, to practice preventative medicine). Herbs such as ginkgo biloba and panax ginseng have been recommended by TCM practitioners for this purpose for nearly 5,000 years.

Acupuncture

As part of a holistic approach to mental and physical health, TCM has long used the art of acupuncture in conjunction with herbal remedies. The underlying principle is the flow of vital energy, or "qi" (pronounced "chee") along defined paths in the body known as meridians. If the natural flow of energy is disrupted, pain or illness results. Placing fine needles into the blocked meridian reestablishes the qi so that the body can be healed by a healthy energy flow. Elaborate maps of the meridian lines of the body were developed to determine the appropriate acupuncture points to affect the healing process.

Because this theory is not reconcilable with our modern understanding of neurologic, chemical, and hormonal communication throughout the body, acupuncture was summarily dismissed as a placebo remedy by Western medicine for many years until the benefits in certain situations seemed consistent and reproducible.

A recent National Institutes of Health (NIH) Consensus Development Conference reviewed the literature on acupuncture since 1970 and listened to the opinions from experts in the field. They concluded that "acupuncture may be useful as an adjunct treatment or an acceptable alternative" for a variety of conditions. The group found the efficacy of acupuncture was particularly strong for management of postoperative and chemotherapy-induced nausea and vomiting and postoperative dental pain. There was also support for acupuncture in managing nausea in pregnancy and in relieving the pain of menstrual cramps, tennis elbow, and fibromyalgia. The consensus panel approved of acupuncture as an adjunct or alternative treatment in stroke rehabilitation, addiction, asthma, and for patients with a variety of painful conditions including headache, myofacial pain, osteoarthritis, lower back pain, and carpal tunnel syndrome.

We now think acupuncture may have positive benefits for muscle spasm by the release of negatively charged ions that accumulate in damaged muscles and cause spasms. It is also widely accepted that the microtrauma caused by the needle insertion triggers the release of pain-reducing substances in the brain called endorphins. The fact that acupuncture points tend to be in areas of decreased electrical resistance may also be part of the scientific basis for the beneficial effects. It is interesting that many of the conditions known to cause depression or be caused by depression (such as chronic pain, fibromyalgia, and carpal tunnel syndrome) are helped by acupuncture. These positive benefits for the reduction of pain and muscle tension go a long way in allowing the patient to become relaxed and in a more positive emotional and mental state. And, of course, we should never underestimate the healing power of an empathetic practitioner who has a hands-on involvement with the patient in treatment.

Aromatherapy

The sense of smell is carried by the first cranial nerve, called the olfactory nerve, which originates in the cribiform plate in the nose and communicates directly to the olfactory area of the brain. This area, in turn, sends signals to the hypothalamus and limbic areas, including the amygdala. As discussed on page 95, this is the seat of our emotional response, and we should not be surprised that it is influenced strongly by the sense of smell.

Many of you may have noticed how a certain smell may suddenly bring back a happy or painful memory. Or, you may have a sudden sense of deja vu without remembering exactly where you have smelled a fragrance before. The smell of your own bed and your significant other's skin and hair as you snuggle in bed gives you an immediate sense of calm and comfort. When you are away from home, you may have difficulty achieving the same degree of relaxation in a hotel bed.

Aromatherapy uses the essential oils of a variety of herb and plant extracts. When warmed gently over a small candle flame, the liquid oil evaporates into gas that the patient then inhales and smells. Research has shown that different essential oils have very different effects on our brains and emotions. Jasmine seems to increase brain waves in the beta range that come from the front of the brain, causing increased alertness and work productivity. Lavender, which increases alpha waves in the back of the brain, is well known to induce drowsiness and relaxation.

Insomniacs have been shown to sleep better if their rooms are scented with lavender. The mood-altering therapies that have been shown to be of benefit for stress, anxiety, insomnia, and nervous tension include lavender, chamomile, neroli, bergamot, sweet marjoram, and ylang-ylang. A hot lavender bath, in which several drops of the oil are placed in a tub full of warm water, may be better than a sedative in calming your nerves, relaxing your muscles, and preparing your mind for rest.

Homeopathy

Dr. Samuel Hahnemann was a famous German physician in the 1800s who gave up his successful medical practice because he saw that patients eventually came back with a new problem even though they felt better if he suppressed their symptoms with medicines. He figured that modern medical science's ability to suppress an illness in the body was causing the new ailment to surface because the patient's body had not been allowed to overcome the original disease. He went back to the drawing board and found that many physicians before him, including Hippocrates and Paracelsus, were using an entirely different method in following the natural law of similars. This principle states, "let likes be cured by likes."

In the words of Hippocrates, "Through the like, disease is produced, and through the application of the like, it is cured." Hahnemann created the name from the Greek words *homeo* ,which means similar, and *pathy*, meaning disease or suffering. Homeopathy holds that very small doses of "similars," or something that in a higher dose would cause similar symptoms as the disease itself, will induce a healing response by which the body will correct or cure the underlying disease condition. In Western medicine, we use a similar philosophy when giving allergy shots. By giving small doses of the substance that causes the allergy, the body becomes desensitized to the allergic substance (known as the allergen) so that it no longer triggers an allergic reaction.

Dr. Hahnemann developed hundreds of remedies for nearly every ailment imaginable through somewhat scientific experiments on volunteers. These experiments are recorded in his *Repertory of Homeopathics*. In the cholera epidemic in Europe during the 1830s, Dr. Hahnemann's patients had a 20 percent death rate, compared to the 50 percent death rate for patients of his medical colleagues. Hahnemann administered a homeopathic remedy that would cause cholera-like symptoms in patients without bringing on the full-fledged disease itself.

Although homeopathy is primarily a German medical tradition with ancient Greek roots, it is also used extensively in France, Brazil, Argentina, and Mexico. Forty percent of European doctors are HMDs (Homeopathic Medical Doctors), 70 percent of doctors in India are HMDs, and the physician for the Queen of England and the Royal Family is an HMD. There are more than 2,000 different homeopathic remedies that are available without a prescription. They are not only used by the HMDs, but also medical doctors, dentists, acupuncturists, chiropractors, and even veterinarians.

A study in the September 20, 1997, issue of the medical journal *Lancet*, 89 studies of homeopathic remedies were analyzed. It was shown that the remedies were almost two-and-a-half times more effective than placebo. These remedies are derived from plants, herbs, animal and mineral sources. There has never been, in 200 years, a homeopathic remedy that has been recalled or taken off the market for adverse effects.

As far as anxiety and depression are concerned, a homeopathic physician may recommend one or more of the following after taking a detailed history of symptoms:

❑ **Ignatia:** For worry, insomnia, fear, and emotional stress.
❑ **Gelsemium:** For stage fright, fear of public speaking, apprehension, trembling, and diarrhea.
❑ **Aconite:** For anxiety, dizziness, and stress headache.
❑ **Pulsatilla:** For insomnia, anxiety, and fearfulness.
❑ **Arsenicum album:** For worry, emotional exhaustion, and fatigue.
❑ **Coffea cruda:** For jittery nerves, racing thoughts, and mental exhaustion.

There are two homeopathic remedies that are being produced by Lehning Laboratories in France: *Sleep Ease* (a nonaddictive sleep aid) and *Anti-Anxiety* (a nonsedating anxiety remedy for daytime use). They are popular in Europe and are now being distributed in the United States.

According to Dr. Roger Morrison of the Hahnemann Medical Clinic in Point Richmond, California, "In acute disease, relief can occur in a few hours or in a day or two. In chronic diseases, however, improvement is slow and gradual, typically taking as much as three months to a few years, depending on the severity and duration of the disease and the previous use of standard medicines."

To the experience of many American physicians, the public has an attention span of two minutes and the patience to match. Some patients complain if they haven't felt any relief within 15 minutes of taking a pill. They want years of self-abuse with drinking, smoking, and overeating to be cured within a matter of hours or days. These are falsely high expectations for modern medicine. Take to heart, instead, the rule of Dr. Jack Ritchason in his *The Vitamin and Health Encyclopedia*, "Nothing heals in the human body in less than three months, and then add one month for every year that you have been sick."

There are other cautions to be observed when using homeopathic medicines, as pointed out by Dr. Morrison "It is important not to eat, drink, smoke, or use toothpaste for 15 minutes before and after taking the remedy. Remedies should be stored at room temperature in a dry, dark place. They should not be exposed to direct sunlight or strong odors."

In addition, several things can interfere with the effectiveness of homeopathic medicines. "Antidotes" block the intended effect of the medicine and render it ineffective. Common antidotes include coffee (decaf and regular), camphor, menthol, Ben Gay, tiger balm, tea tree oil, skin cleansers, cough lozenges, lip balm, and some Chinese candies. "Suppression" occurs if the person takes a standard allopathic drug or herbal remedy designed to suppress the symptom, which, in the theory of homeopathic medicine, weakens the patient's natural ability to fight the illness.

Vitamins and supplements

Vitamins and minerals generally work to help support the body in performing its natural functions. The theory is that these supplements are depleted by stress, poor dietary intake, poor intestinal absorption, exposure to pollutants, pain, illness — and even prescription medications. To help the body maintain optimal health, supplemental intake of various nutrients are helpful.

Few physicians discourage the use of reasonable amounts of vitamins and supplements in individuals who are not coping well with stress, are particularly vulnerable because of alcohol or cigarette smoking, have poor sleeping and eating habits, are born with poor immune resistance, or have other medical problems. Certain vitamins are mentioned repeatedly in the literature for improving the body's response to stress, as well as calming anxiety, insomnia and irritability, and relieving depression and fatigue. Here is a brief list of vitamins and supplements thought to be helpful with various problems:

❑ **Anxiety, irritability, and insomnia:** Niacin (vitamin B3), vitamin B6, vitamin B15, folic acid, choline, L-tryptophan, vitamin A, beta carotene, chromium, inositol, B-complex, calcium and magnesium, silicon, multiple vitamin/mineral supplement, and manganese.

- ❏ **Depression and fatigue:** Vitamin B12 (preferably given by injection), B-complex, calcium and magnesium, flower essence, pyridoxine (B6), thiamine (B1), niacin (B3), choline, chromium, vanadium, zinc, lecithin, iodine, potassium, essential fatty acids, vitamin C, L-tyrosine, folic acid, and inositol.
- ❏ **Stress:** B-complex (especially B2, B5, B6, and B15), folic acid, vitamin C with bioflavonoids, vitamin E, calcium, magnesium, lecithin, phosphorus, Bach flower remedy, zinc potassium, and L-tyrosine.
- ❏ **Bipolar disorder:** Amino acids such as L-tyrosine and L-taurine, B-complex, mineral complex, iodine, chromium, vanadium, B1, B2, B6, B12, vitamin C with bioflavonoids, calcium and magnesium, potassium, and essential fatty acids.

Vitamins and supplements used to fight stress

Vitamin B1 (thiamine)

Thiamine is necessary for the body to make use of its carbohydrate intake. Deficiency can lead to brain dysfunction known as Wernicke's encephalopathy. Milder symptoms include anxiety, insomnia, agitation, mood swings, fatigue, muscle weakness, heart palpitations, and confusion. In the diet, thiamine may be found in whole grains, oatmeal, bran, most vegetables, peanuts, legumes (beans and peas), and oranges. Known as a "stress vitamin," the need for thiamine increases with trauma, illness, surgery, pregnancy, nursing, as well as alcohol and nicotine addictions. It has also helped those with seasickness. Its main claim to fame is strengthening the nervous system and improving mental attitude.

Vitamin B2 (riboflavin)

Riboflavin helps the body digest fats, proteins, and carbohydrates in order to utilize the energy from these nutrient sources. It also helps convert amino acids into neurotransmitters needed for normal brain function, necessary in the production of red blood cells (for oxygen transport from the lungs to the tissues) and antibody formation (for the immune system to fight infection). Deficiency can lead to hair loss, blurred vision, depression, dizziness, and skin irritation. Good sources for vitamin B2 are spinach, dairy products, broccoli, green leafy vegetables, fish, eggs, and poultry.

Vitamin B3 (niacin)

Niacin is necessary for a healthy nervous system and proper brain function. A deficiency of this vitamin has been associated with negative personality changes. It has been used by some practitioners to aid in the treatment of a variety of mental disorders, including anxiety, nervousness, and depression. The body can produce its own B3 if there is enough B1, B2, and B6. Supplements of niacin commonly cause a transient flushing and itching of the skin. Good sources include tuna, chicken breast, fortified breads and cereals, wheat germ, dates, figs, prunes, broccoli, tomatoes, and carrots.

Vitamin B5 (pantothenic acid)

Vitamin B5 is necessary for the production of a variety of hormones needed to fight stress and is involved in the production of antibodies as well. It helps convert fats, carbohydrates, and proteins to usable energy. Good sources include mushrooms, salmon, peanuts, whole grains, chicken, wheat germ, broccoli, green vegetables, and tomatoes.

Vitamin B6 (pyridoxine)

Vitamin B6 is needed by the body to make serotonin, the neurotransmitter most closely linked with regulating anxiety and depression. Recent studies have shown it to be especially helpful for women who suffer from PMS. A deficiency of B6 can cause irritability, dizziness, depression, and anxiety. Good sources include milk, soy beans, nuts, wheat bran and wheat germ, cantaloupe, bananas, leafy green vegetables, peas, salmon, and cod. People with Parkinson's disease on the drug Levodopa should not take B6 supplements.

A good quality B-complex supplement taken up to twice a day should provide all your B-vitamin needs, especially during times of high stress.

Vitamin B12 (cyanocobalamin)

This is actually a coenzyme needed to metabolize fats and carbohydrates. Vitamin B12 also protects nerves from damage and promotes normal growth. Some forms of dementia have been linked to low levels of this vitamin in the bloodstream. Those who lack an enzyme made in the stomach that is needed to absorb vitamin B12 from the diet get a form of anemia known as pernicious anemia, which must be corrected with intramuscular shots of B12. I commonly give one to five cc (cubic centimeters) of B12 injection to those with viral illnesses and general fatigue to help with energy level and general sense of well-being. Good sources include clams, crab, tuna, salmon, oysters, dairy products, and tofu.

Vitamin E

Like vitamin C, vitamin E is an antioxidant and is thought to help prevent heart disease and cancer. There is some evidence that vitamin E may slow down the aging process by prolonging the life span of cells in the body. Vitamin E may also help protect the body from a number of toxins and carcinogens, including heavy metals (mercury, lead), nitrites, benzene, cigarette smoke, and air pollution. Vitamin E speeds up tissue regeneration and reduces scar tissue, especially if applied directly to the healing wound. The daily dose should be 400 IU (international units).

Mineral supplementation

Several minerals are important in the production of brain neurotransmitters. The depletion of these minerals is caused by stress, alcohol, and caffeine. It is a good idea to take a daily supplement of magnesium, copper, chromium, manganese, and selenium a day. Researchers at the University College of Swansea in Wales found that those who took 100 mcg (micrograms) of selenium per day felt stronger emotionally, with less anxiety and depression, than those who were not given the supplement. Selenium is a potent antioxidant that protects the immune system. It promotes energy and stamina and is very helpful in combination with vitamin E. Selenium is often deficient in the diet due to low levels in the soil and poor eating habits. It can be found in wheat germ, asparagus, mushrooms, tuna, lobster, crab, clams, and oysters. A daily multimineral supplement should cover your dose.

5HTP

5-hydroxytryptophan (5HTP) is created in the body from the amino acid tryptophan. 5HTP is then used in the process of creating serotonin. Because of its ability to easily cross the blood-brain barrier and enter the brain from the bloodstream, taking supplemental doses of 5HTP ultimately increases brain serotonin levels.

The 5HTP sold in stores comes from the *Griffonia* seed, the product of an African tree grown mostly in Ghana and the Ivory Coast. 5HTP became available in the United States in 1994 as an over-the-counter supplement. In his book *5-Htp, Nature's Serotonin Solution*, Ray Sahelian, M.D., gives a detailed look at the supplement, its uses, benefits, and side effects. Like many of the SSRIs, the lists of disorders helped by 5HTP is long, including weight control, depression, anxiety disorders, insomnia, fibromyalgia, PMS, and migraine headaches. Doses and dosing regimens are variable depending on the disorder you are treating. The supplement is considered safe and is generally well tolerated.

DHEA

Dihydroepiandrosterone (DHEA) is an adrenal and gonadal hormone has been shown in some studies to have mood-elevating qualities. It has been studied in the elderly to test effects on mental functioning. It was shown to improve vitality, memory, concentration, and other cognitive factors in many subjects. DHEA serves to regulate hormone balance and is a precursor to estrogen and progesterone. Some have claimed that it helps their sex drive because some of the DHEA is eventually converted into testosterone in the body. Others have noticed improvement in sleep patterns and their ability to cope with stress. Because levels of this hormone naturally decrease with age, it is usually recommended for those in their midforties and older. Did DHEA really help Mark McGwire hit so many home runs in 1998-1999? It didn't hurt.

The maximum daily dose for long-term use is 5 mg per day. Overuse of DHEA can cause acne, hair loss, and heart palpitations. Use of DHEA (or pregnenolone) should be done only under medical supervision and after a complete medical evaluation.

SAM-e

SAM-e (also spelled SAMe and Sam-E in various sources) is the popular name for S-adrenosyl-methionine. It has been used for many years throughout Europe as a dietary supplement, particularly in Italy, where its antidepressant effects were first reported in 1973. During the last year, SAM-e has become increasingly popular in the United States. Subsequently, SAM-e has been studied for its antiinflammatory effects and its usefulness as an antioxidant.

SAM-e is produced mainly in the liver and is an active form of the amino acid methionine, which is found in most body fluids and tissues. The production of SAM-e in the body requires folic acid and vitamin B12. It has been found that individuals with liver disease, heart disease, and depression have lower levels of SAM-e. Alcoholics are usually deficient in the vitamins necessary to make SAM-e.

The monoamine brain neurotransmitters (including serotonin, dopamine, and norepinephrine) are built with the help of SAM-e through its donation of a methyl group to those brain chemicals. Comparison studies have been conducted between SAM-e and classic tricyclic antidepressants such as Elavil, Norpramin, and Sinequan. These studies suggest that SAM-e may work faster than these drugs, with fewer side effects and equal effectiveness. SAM-e comes in 200 mg strength tablets and can be found in most drug stores and health food/nutrition centers. It should be stored in a dry, dark place. The usual dose of SAM-e for depression is 200 to 800 mg twice a day.

Pregnenolone

As the parent hormone of DHEA, pregnenolone understandably has similar effects. Users claim enhanced mood and alertness, along with improvement in vision and hearing. Again, the regular daily dosage should not exceed 5 mg, and side effects of overuse are similar to those of DHEA.

Phytochemicals

There is much concern these days about not getting enough vine-ripened fruits and vegetables. Fruits and vegetables are often picked early to be shipped to the supermarket and are allowed to ripen in boxes or in the produce department warehouse. This may prevent the production of hundreds — and possibly thousands — of phytochemicals that are manufactured in the fruits and vegetables during the final stage of ripening while still on the vine. These chemicals may have antioxidant and disease-fighting properties more powerful than those in vitamins, and include limonenes in citrus fruits, indoles and isothiocynates in broccoli, flavones in dried beans, genistein in soybeans, and flavonoids in almost all fruits and vegetables.

Many of these compounds are thought to neutralize free radicals, unstable molecules that bind to cellular components and damage them. These free radicals are created in the body during times of stress and exposure to ultraviolet radiation, cigarette smoke, car fumes, or other pollutants and toxins. Their destructive power may accelerate aging and contribute to the development of heart disease and cancer. Phytochemicals stabilize free radicals and prevent this damage. If you cannot eat five to nine servings a day of fruits and vegetables, you might consider a phytochemical substitute. Pharmaceutical grade extracts, such as those by Juice Plus, can be taken once or twice daily.

For those who resist female hormone replacement at menopause, it may be wise to consume foods that are rich in phytoestrogens, or plant estrogens. For some women, these plant sources may be adequate to reduce or stop hot flashes, as well as the anxiety, depression, and irritability caused by estrogen deficiency. Plants high in phytoestrogens include yams, soybeans, flaxseeds, kale, millet, bok choy, and mustard greens. We don't know if these sources have the additional benefits in preventing heart disease and osteoporosis, which has been proven with pharmaceutical estrogen replacement, because research in this area has not yet been done.

Summing up for now

The old saying, "Try it—it can't hurt you," does not apply to vitamin, mineral, or other supplements any more than it applies to prescription drugs. Even the long, safe use of a particular substance in another culture or our own does not guarantee that it is right for you and your condition. Therefore, combine your own research with the advice of a knowledgeable health professional before stocking up on alternative treatments for anxiety, panic, and depression.

Barbara... A.P.D., Public Places, and Performance

Let me take you to two special circles of emotional hell reserved for people like me with A.P.D. symptoms. The first is wherever a large group is assembled, where leaving unexpectedly is awkward or impolite, and where the people around you might be aware of your display of discomfort. These places can include theatres, church or synagogue, concert halls, lectures, and the like. For some of us, the list expands to arenas, stadiums, business meetings, and civic gatherings.

The second pressure cooker is made up of the broad range of performance situations where others are depending on you, you have to "keep going" no matter what, and there's no backup plan to rely upon. The examples from my list of horror moments are many, but here are a few:

I had foolishly agreed to driving a carload of Girl Scouts from my daughter's troop to a theme park some 30 miles away. Other parents were also driving their cars and were moving down the freeway in a caravan. The whole time, I was thinking: "Uh-oh, what if my panic starts to build and take over? What if a sudden run of heart palpitations occurs while I'm driving these kids? If I have to pull over on the freeway or take an unplanned detour to the nearest offramp, what do I say to the kids or to their parents? What if I can't continue to drive for an hour or more while I get myself back together? What if I'm able to gut it out and actually get to the theme park, but then fall apart in complete exhaustion as I try to lead my little brood of kids around the park? What do I say? What will the other parents say about me?"

Second example: I was alone, driving my car during rush hour across a long bridge (or, if you wish, substitute a tunnel, busy freeway, or a similar "no exit" experience). There's no emergency lane, no room to pull over. I have to keep going at the prevailing speed of traffic. If I slow down or have to stop due to panic, traffic will immediately back up behind me, horns will blow, and within minutes, an emergency vehicle will pull up beside my stopped car to find out what the trouble is. As I sit there in the driver's seat, my face will be white as a sheet and my heart will be beating like crazy. What exactly do I say? "Sorry, my good man, but I'm having a full-fledged panic attack. Perhaps you've read of panic disorder in *Redbook* or *Reader's Digest*? Now you get to see it live. No, don't call an ambulance. Just give me about half an hour blocking traffic here on the bridge and then I'll be off again on my way home to tell my family how my day was."

Here is a final example: I was on a cruise, recommended by my doctor to soothe my nerves. I crossed over the gang plank with my husband. The huge boat began to move from shore and the familiar, awful feelings swept over me, accompanied by panicked thoughts: "I'm stuck on this thing no matter what for the next seven days. There's no doctor on board. If I experience panic, my only refuge is that closet of a room, which in itself could drive me nuts. No porthole. No room to breathe. Yet to feel anxiety and panic out on deck in public is unthinkable. What do I say to people passing by if they notice I'm in distress? What about my poor, long-suffering husband who has looked forward to this cruise as his only vacation this year? Doesn't he deserve better? Do I have to ruin everything for him as well as for myself?"

If the cruise scenario doesn't click with your experience, feel free to substitute a bus or train trip, a guided walk through a museum or large garden, or any circumstance where you get on, you can't stop, and you have to keep it together.

9 | What Can I Do on My Own to Fight Anxiety, Panic, and Depression?

The theme of previous chapters is to seek professional guidance before diagnosing your own ills or inventing ways to treat them. That being said, there's much you can do in your daily life to support good health and speed recovery from anxiety, panic, and depression—or prevent them in the first place.

The basics

Eating, sleeping, breathing, and drinking fluids are the basic natural needs of the body that must be met to sustain life and provide the body the ability for healing. Beyond this, we can exercise, laugh, enjoy our sexual capacities, commune with nature, work in the garden, play with a pet, experience and appreciate art and music, work on various meditation and visualization techniques, talk to a trusted friend, seek professional counseling, try hypnotherapy, cognitive behavioral therapy, or biofeedback strategies, work on developing an ethical code of conduct, or explore a spiritual or religious belief system to sustain us in good times and bad.

These are natural strategies in the sense that healing comes from within. It springs from an emotional will to heal and better oneself rather than depend on some external drug, herb, supplement, vitamin, or aroma to make us well. Ultimately, only this type of personal involvement in the healing process can allow the individual to truly rise above and overcome anxiety, panic, and depression.

Facing anxiety and depression

Perhaps one of most obvious (but least heeded) pieces of advice is to deal with your problems rather than just running from them. It takes courage and sometimes even a spiritual revelation for us to look at ourselves without flinching. In this evaluation of our attitudes and behavior, we may find that we ourselves have the problem—not "everyone else."

Sometimes we see our problems clearly but we are so paralyzed by anxiety and depression that we don't know which direction to move or where to start. Nor do we have the energy in these states to make the first move. Indecision is a common symptom of emotional dysfunction and is often the first and biggest stumbling block in recovering from these disorders.

Here's where a clear, specific plan of action comes to the rescue. Yogi Berra once said, "If you come to a fork in the road, take it." It often doesn't matter which road you choose—the only wrong decision is no decision at all. Whether you stay where you are or move across the country, whether you leave the relationship or stay in it, whether you take the job or don't—just make up your mind and act. You will always have options as life unfolds. In a way, life is a series of decisions, and when decisions stop, life stands still and stagnates.

Identify the source of your stress by making a list of problem areas in your life. Then, make a plan of how you will address each problem and work on its resolution. Now take your plan to those you trust—a friend, a family member, your doctor, or your spiritual leader—and get some feedback as you form your plan of action. Get professional advice (from a lawyer, accountant, financial planner, etc.) on those items that require information or skills that you don't have. Review the list every day to make sure you are moving forward in resolving the stressful issues on your list. It may be extremely difficult, anxiety provoking, or even depressing to have to face these things. But you must face them. They do not go away by themselves.

One patient was so overwhelmed by depression that she has not done her laundry, paid her bills, or washed a dish in a month. Here, the plan was simple: Get out of bed, put the dirty clothes in a big pile and separate the whites from the colors, take the loads down to the Laundromat, buy some soap, obtain some quarters...you get the message.

In accomplishing your plan, take one day at a time. Don't concentrate on all problems at once. Work on the most basic problems first (food, clothing, shelter, etc.), and you will find the situation improving slowly. Ironically, we have all produced many plans in our lives for remodeling or redecorating our homes, restoring a car, revamping the garden, or settling details for a vacation. If we spent the same time and energy in dealing with personal issues and obstacles, we would be farther along the road to health.

Try not to let others take over completely in "helping" you with problems. No one can take over our lives for us and our problems won't disappear unless we take steps to correct them ourselves. Should we accept help? Of course. But the best kind of help from friends, relatives, and loved ones is the kind of help that encourages our own best efforts. It's no act of kindness to allow a depressed friend to lie in bed while we take over all his or her life responsibilities. Nor is it helpful in the long run to "help" an anxious friend or spouse sidestep every possible challenge or stress presented by daily living.

Letting go

So you have done what you can. You have faced the problems, made a plan of action, and started implementing it day by day. You're taking responsibility and control of your life. Now it's time to let go of the things that you can't control. It's time to let go of the destructive habits and behaviors that hold you back and get you into trouble repeatedly. It's time to really experience life, enjoy being yourself, and find true meaning and purpose. We hope that the remainder of this book will encourage you on that journey.

Here are a few brief recommendations:

1. Live in the present. Let go of past regrets and future worries. Enjoy what the present moment has to offer.

2. Simplify your life and focus on the things that matter most. Let go of the time-consuming, hectic, and unrealistic strategies for reducing stress and work on simple techniques.

3. Let go of the demands you make on yourself. Don't expect to get well overnight. Natural healing, much like the natural growth of a tree, takes place in its own time and without being forced.

4. Accept yourself as you are. Let go of the fantasy of who you thought you would or should be. Let go of worrying about your imperfections. Self-acceptance and self-love are accomplished by looking outside of yourself and seeing yourself in relation to others.

5. Expect setbacks — don't use them as an excuse to despair and revert to old bad habits. You will have good and bad days, but if you keep faith in healing power within yourself you will climb in a positive direction.

6. Let go of the habit of hurrying.

7. Look for sources of inspiration and follow them. Let go of things you are not passionate about and follow the things you are.

8. Let go of that uptight person inside of you who can't have fun or live joyfully. Enjoy nature. Enjoy friends. Take a walk in the woods, swim in a lake, watch the sunset, or smell the roses.

9. Turn off your pager or cellular phone and take a break. In the words of Leonardo Da Vinci, "Every now and then go away, even briefly, and have a little relaxation. For when you come back to your work, your judgment will be surer; to remain constantly at work will cause you to lose power."

10. Relax. This is really a process of letting go, and it cannot be forced. The relaxation response, studied and written about extensively by Dr. Herbert Benson, can be attained through a variety of meditations and can also be taught through bio-feedback techniques.

11. Be quiet. Let go of your compulsion to have the last word. Healing cannot occur until you stop talking and fussing.

12. Free your mind from the clutter and congestion of meaningless trivial pursuits and concerns.

13. Imagine and visualize a more fulfilled and harmonious existence. Let go of your fear of the future and your pessimistic foreboding.

14. Let go of intolerance, hatred, or racism—it poisons your growth as a human being.

15. Sex (including masturbation) is healthy—as long as it doesn't make you late for work.

16. Let go of blaming and looking for excuses. Take full responsibility for yourself.

17. Live fully. Let go of the notion that you are weak and fragile. You aren't.

18. Let go of worry. Mark Twain wrote, "Worry is like a rocking chair. It goes back and forth but gets you nowhere." If a worrisome thought is nagging you that something bad is going to happen, ask yourself, "What if this happens," and then "Well then, so what? What's the worst that could happen? Do I have control over it anyway?" Another technique called thought-stopping was at least present from Biblical times. Jesus, in Matthew 4:10 (NIV), rebuffs the temptations of Satan in the wilderness by saying, "Away from me!" By saying something similar to a worrisome thought that disturbs your peace of mind, you can often break the bondage of the worry habit.

19. Let go of failure. Sir Winston Churchill said, "Success is going from failure to failure without loss of enthusiasm." Nothing is gained without the risk of failure, so don't worry about it. At least you tried. Now get back on the horse and try again.

Eating

Because we depend on eating to sustain our earthly existence, it can affect us in profound ways. For example, Christian religious rituals lift elements of bread and wine as sacred symbols, which are then given as nourishment for the soul. Many of us feel secure and alive and happy as long as food is involved. The happy memories of the family around the dinner table, the picnics and the barbecues, the dinner invitation from cherished friends, the intimate table for two at a favorite restaurant...these are the pictures that stand out in our mental photo album.

Because food affects us emotionally, it is not surprising that anxiety and depression often lead to eating disorders. We may use food to calm our anxiety or overeating in an attempt to feel the calming effects of a high carbohydrate meal. The behavior is repeated through positive reinforcement until we have gained so much weight that we have something else to be depressed about.

Other times, our anxiety turns off our appetite and food is the furthest thing from our minds. The very thought of food in this state of mind can bring feelings of nausea.

Lastly, we may set ourselves up to be unnecessarily vulnerable to anxiety and depression by not following some basic rules of good nutrition. As Dr. Art Ulene, M.D., has admonished, "A poor diet plus vitamins is still a poor diet." One should eat a variety of foods every day in reasonable portions. Don't overeat or undereat. Many national health organizations advise moving toward a vegetarian diet, including whole grains, beans and other legumes, fresh fruits and vegetables, and low-fat or nonfat dairy products. For those who like a little meat, skinless poultry and fish may be added. We would probably do well if beef and pork, like birthday cake, were reserved for that very infrequent special occasion.

Thirty-eight percent of new vegetarians said they felt more alert and vigorous, and less tired and stressed, seven months after eliminating meat from the diet. Dr. Dean Edell was an avid vegetarian for many years before taking the stand that moderation in all things is the best policy.

It is a good general rule to cut down on animal fats and sweets. Avoid chemical residues by washing your fruits and vegetables. Do not rely on vitamin supplements to provide you with the nutrition needed for good physical and emotional health. As with many things in life, the art of eating involves a balance of nutritional, emotional, and spiritual needs that must be achieved for the optimal health and well-being of the individual.

Sleeping

Sleeping problems are one of the most common complaints in people suffering from emotional illness. Sixty percent of those with major depression have insomnia. For physicians, insomnia is "priority number one" to be resolved, whether it came before or after the onset of depression, if the other treatments are to be successful.

Short-term insomnia is defined as occurring one to two nights per week over a three week period. It is estimated to occur in most adults (85 percent) each year in the United States. Chronic insomnia, which is experienced by 10 to 33 percent of adults in the United States, persists for more than three weeks and can have multiple causes, including physical and emotional disorders. Some people have the condition of sleep apnea and aren't aware that their sleep is interrupted over and over during the course of the night.

The sleep deprivation caused by chronic insomnia is the number-one cause of traffic accidents and fatalities in the United States. For this reason alone, it should be considered a potentially life-threatening condition. The first step in dealing with chronic insomnia is to get a thorough evaluation from your primary care physician. Once the causes of the sleep problem have been identified, issues of sleep health and medical and alternative options should be discussed. The goal is to resolve the sleep deficiency in a way which is safe and does not interfere with other treatments.

Sleep loss may be the actual reason a person develops depression in the first place. Research has shown that those with insomnia are four times more likely to develop depression. If you have a co-worker who is developing a depressed mood, yawning frequently during the day, and having periods of impaired work performance, he or she may have been experiencing a bout of chronic insomnia. The medications to treat depression may also cause or contribute to insomnia. This is particularly true with the SSRI fluoxetine.

The first strategy in approaching insomnia is to review basic principles of sleep health. Here are some basic guidelines:

1. Keep a regular schedule of when you go to bed and when you get up.
2. Avoid afternoon naps.
3. Do your exercise in the morning, not late in the day.
4. Avoid alcohol and caffeine within six hours of bedtime. (Have your wine or beer with lunch.)
5. The bedroom is for sleep and sex. Don't read, watch TV, do paperwork, answer the phone, have arguments, or do anything stressful in the sleep environment.
6. Make sure the bedroom is quiet and comfortable. If you live in a noisy area, get something to create some "white noise," such as a fan.
7. Go to bed in a relaxed mood. If you're not relaxed, consider eating a snack high in carbohydrates, such as grains, legumes, pasta, bread, vegetables, fruits, or a bowl of cereal.
8. Don't lie in bed awake, thinking and worrying. Get up and leave the bedroom, go to the bathroom, eat a snack, or watch part of the late-night movie. When you feel sleepy and relaxed, go back to the bedroom.

After sleep health has been addressed, the patient may want to consider trying some alternative sleep aids before resorting to medications. Herbs shown to be helpful in this regard are kava kava, valerian, hops, passion flower, chamomile, and others (discussed on pages 159-168). Ask your herbalist for a recommendation. Supplements, such as melatonin and 5HTP, are also helpful for some individuals. Marketed as a dietary supplement, melatonin has been shown to improve sleep. However, the purity of the products available and adverse effects are not well known. It is available in a number of forms (tablets, time-release capsules, under-the-tongue lozenges, liquid extract, and tea) and is generally taken at a dose range between 0.3 to 1 mg. Higher dosages may cause morning grogginess or vivid dreaming.

Dr. Ray Sahelian has found that insomnia is best treated by polytherapy. He writes, "By alternating different natural supplements, and even prescription pills when needed, one would run a lower risk of tolerance, and, one hopes, a lower risk of side effects." Aromatherapy or a hot lavender bath may be other helpful options to get into a relaxed mood for sleep. You may also try one of the over-the-counter homeopathic remedies discussed in the section on homeopathy.

Medications from your doctor or over-the-counter preparations are divided into several groups:

1. Antihistamines: The two antihistamines approved by the FDA as "sleep-aids" are diphenhydramine and doxylamine. They are frequently used in the elderly because of general safety. However, it is dangerous to operate motor vehicles or heavy machinery after taking them. In fact, it is illegal (at least in California) to drive under the influence of these substances. Possible adverse effects include dry mouth, constipation, nervousness, and restlessness in some individuals.

2. Antidepressants: These have been discussed earlier, so I will just mention briefly those drugs used routinely to improve sleep in depressed and anxious patients.

❑ *Tricyclics.* Amitriptyline (Elavil) and doxepin (Sinequan) are commonly used in low doses because of their sedative properties. Long-term doxepin treatment was shown to increase the brain's production of melatonin. In the elderly especially, side effects can be a problem (urinary retention, constipation, dry mouth, and blurred vision).

❑ *Trazodone* (Desyrel). It has few drug interactions and can be mixed with other antidepressants. It is not lethal in overdose unless combined with alcohol. It may cause daytime sedation.

❑ *Nefazadone* (Serzone). Increases sleep efficiency and reduces number of awakenings, with no sexual dysfunction. May cause next day drowsiness.

❑ *Mirtazapine* (Remeron). This very sedating, new-generation antidepressant frequently causes weight gain. Higher doses cause *less* sedation than lower doses.

3. Benzodiazepines: Relatively safe and effective, these drugs are the mainstay of pharmacological treatment of insomnia. Because of tolerance and dependency issues, use should be limited to one month and only used for difficult cases. Temazepam (Restoril), as well as Dalmane, Halcion, Xanax, and Valium are examples of benzodiazepine sleeping medications. They are designed to get into the bloodstream quickly and get out fast enough to prevent morning sedation.

4. Other: Zolpidem (Ambien) is the newest of the hypnotic agents and is available in 5 and 10 mg doses, taken at bedtime. It is very effective, causes little morning sedation, and is not as addictive as the benzodiazepines. However, tolerance (needing more) and dependence can occur. One caution is to be careful if you are taking this drug in an unfamiliar situation where you might be awakened, such as in an airplane where you need to make a transfer in the middle of the night, because you may be disoriented and confused.

Music

Music powerfully affects our mood and emotions and reduces stress, as shown by many research studies. Music has been shown to reduce the levels of stress hormones, blood pressure, breathing rate, and the peristaltic contractions in the intestines. As you will read in the section on meditation, it is used as part of healing meditation for pain and anxiety control in cancer patients. It can make us feel like sleeping, laughing, crying, singing, making love, marching, or dancing. It helps us forget our worries, puts our fears on hold, or have the courage to charge into battle. It allows us to release painful emotions, let down our guard, and feel love and closeness towards others.

In a recent interview in *Bon Appetite* magazine, Ray Charles was asked to recall a particularly memorable meal. "I'll never forget the time I met Itzhak Perlman. We were at a studio taping a public service announcement and at some point someone sent out for some barbecue. He loved it as much as I did, and we were there eating and laughing, and when I said, 'Play your fiddle,' he got up and played a little *Georgia* for me."

People who would never otherwise meet, who come from different sides of the track or different sides of the world, are brought together by the universal language of music. Great music is like a mirror that lets us see our inner heart more clearly and appreciate our human experience more profoundly.

Music therapy is becoming increasingly recognized as a valuable tool for calming anxiety and dissipating stress. Many physicians make sure that anyone who visits their offices is greeted by music and interesting artwork. Whether it be a sophisticated symphony or the simple sounds of a waterfall, music touches us deeply.

Exercise

Like it or not, we are born into a physical body that requires regular maintenance and exercise. There is no question about the many benefits of exercise on physical and emotional health. This includes reducing the risks of disease, as well as improved resistance to anxiety and depression. Exercise has been shown to improve mood, immune system functioning, mental alertness and memory, sexual functioning, and digestive functioning. It decreases pain, insomnia, headaches, anxiety, and combats heart disease, obesity, arthritis, emphysema, diabetes, and many other common illnesses.

The most common excuse is "Where will I find the time?" The answer is that you don't really need to. You just need to change how you go about your day. New research indicates that short bursts of exercise can help even the most sedentary people get fit, while helping with stress, anxiety, weight loss, stamina, and improving the cholesterol and triglyceride levels in the bloodstream. In fact, in several studies from Northern Ireland and the University of Pittsburgh, short bursts (two to 10 minutes) of exercise several times a day are preferable to traditional 40- to 60-minute workouts for weight loss and provide equal benefits for blood pressure lowering and decreasing fats in the bloodstream.

So you don't need that evasive 90-minute chunk of time that it takes to get into the work-out clothes, drive to the gym, wait in line for the machines, shower up, and drive home. But you do have two minutes here and there to run up the stairs instead of taking the elevator, run the dog a few times around the block before and after work, play soccer with your kids for 10 minutes in the evening, run up and down the stairs at work for three minutes before lunch, or do short bursts on an exercise bike while talking on the phone or watching TV. Get a punching bag or jump rope and pretend you're Ali getting ready for Frasier. If you have any motivation at all, you should be able to slip in two or three bursts of activity every day.

You might pick a few days a week to get back into your favorite sport. Take tennis or swimming lessons, join a hiking club, get into ballroom and performance dancing, play frisbee with your dog, get a season ticket to your favorite ski resort, get your mountain bike off those hooks in the garage rafters, or wax up your windsurfing board.

There is also good evidence that strength training may be as valuable as aerobic training for weight loss, blood pressure control, and stress reduction. Just 15 minutes two to three times a week may be adequate for great results. Choose five big muscle group areas, such as arms (biceps and triceps), chest (pectoralis majors), shoulders and back (triceps, rhomboids), abdominals, and thighs (quadriceps and hamstrings). Have a weight trainer teach you one exercise for each of these muscles and concentrate on proper technique and form. Always breathe out when you do the exertional part of the exercise and breathe in during the relaxation part. This prevents hernias, undue strain on the muscles, and unhealthy elevations of blood pressure.

You can expect to feel a little stiff and sore the next day, but should not experience sharp pain at any time. If this happens, stop and consult your doctor.

Finally, your body will respond to exercise better if you get into a gentle program of daily stretching. Stretching exercises, along with proper breathing technique, can be especially relaxing and meditative. Plan to spend a few minutes when you get up and a few minutes before going to bed doing a set program of five or six stretches. There are many different disciplines that involve stretching, including yoga and t'ai chi ch'uan, as well as traditional stretches you can learn from a physical therapist or exercise instructor. Dr. Herbert Benson wrote: "There are a number of rhythmic exercises that also elicit the relaxation response. Notable are the various Chinese techniques such as t'ai chi ch'uan. These employ prescribed rhythmic movements with a passive attitude, relaxed muscles, and attention to breathing."

Massage

Massage has been practiced by many different schools, each teaching unique techniques and styles that have long histories and traditions. The goal is to find a style that works for you. For example, you may prefer a slow and methodical working over of each muscle group done the same way each time so your body can relax and let go of the tension. The massage therapist may use aromatherapy and massage oils, as well as soothing musical sounds and dimmed lights. During the massage, try to let your mind drift, even in and out of sleep.

Most surprising about a massage is how you may feel the rest of the day. You may feel in a more pleasant and playful mood than usual, and have more energy throughout the afternoon and evening. Whether you try massage therapy by itself or in combination with traditional Chinese medicine, homeopathy, psychotherapy, or some other form of therapy, you won't be the first to discover the healing power of the human touch.

Pet therapy

Animals, or at least most commonly dogs and cats, have been helping and healing their human keepers for many centuries by lifting the spirits, providing companionship for the lonely, leading the blind, and comforting the bereaved. However, animals have been used in new forms of therapy around the world with astounding results. Dogs have been used in psychiatric therapy sessions for hospitalized patients at Virginia Commonwealth University in Richmond, Virginia. This therapy significantly reduced anxiety in patients with depression, bipolar illness, and schizophrenia. The Dolphin Research Center in Florida found that retarded children were more interactive, verbally communicative, and physically animated when therapy included dolphins, rather than when the children were playing with their favorite toys.

After several weeks of caring for guinea pigs, birds, and other small animals, children with attention deficit disorder improved their grades and behavior better than another group of kids with the same disorder who went canoeing and rock climbing. That study was performed in 1993 by the Devereux Foundation, a treatment facility for troubled kids in Philadelphia. Children with autism, cerebral palsy, Down's syndrome, behavior problems, and difficult personalities seem to respond well to animal therapy. Some credit this to the unconditional love an animal can give, allowing us to relax and be ourselves without fear of judgment or punishment. There is nothing better than therapy that seems like play.

A May 1999 Associated Press story by Mary Pemberton described the value of dogs in helping people with depression, panic disorder, bipolar disorder, and agoraphobia. For instance, dogs can be trained to sense when their master is about to have a panic attack. They recognize changes in scent, breathing rate, and other physical manifestations of an attack early. They respond by leaning against, nuzzling, or standing between their master and a crowd. Many sufferers have found that the calming presence of the dog may stop an oncoming panic attack.

A person with an emotional illness that "substantially limits one or more major life activities," such as leaving the house, can register their dog as a trained service dog under the Americans with Disabilities Act. But even if you don't need an "emotional seeing eye dog" to get out of the house and brave a trip to the supermarket, you still may enjoy unwinding with your pet at the end of a stressful day at the office.

Gardening

It is almost universally satisfying to see the first green leaf bud of a seedling break through the moist soil and turn toward the sun. Every day is a new development if you look closely.

Gardening can get you back in touch with yourself, putting you back in rhythm with nature. Many long-lived senior citizens spend several hours a day tending to plants as if they were their children. The healing powers of horticulture are not lost on the medical field. In 1812, Dr. Benjamin Rush, founding father of the American Psychiatric Association, prescribed gardening to his patients with emotional illness. Over 300 U.S. hospitals have gardens for patient use. The American Horticultural Therapy Association in Gaithersburg, Maryland, has nearly 900 members.

Even if you only have room for a window planterbox or a pottery bowl containing your favorite herbs, getting your fingers dirty seems to trigger our natural healing tendencies.

Comedy and laughter

Long before Patch Adams, laughter was known to help alleviate emotional and physical pain, improve immune system functioning, and help brighten the mood and outlook of those suffering from a variety of illnesses. When feeling stressed out, who doesn't feel better after laughing? Why do we dive into the comedy club or look for comic relief at the movie theater after a high-pressure week at the office? It provides quick and effective relief to laugh at others as well as ourselves. We learn to find humor in what we thought we feared or disliked, including our anxieties and neuroses.

Humor has been found to be a key element in successful marriages and relationships. People who know how to see the lighter side of things are generally able to bounce back from stress easily. Some have theorized that laughter directly triggers the release of brain endorphins that help ease pain and provide a sensation of euphoria and joy. Anyone know a good joke?

Have a beer and watch the game

There is no faster way to get away from your problems, tune out the complaining, and become intellectually and emotionally involved in something totally outside yourself than to get interested in sports. Know the rules. Know the chess game-like cunning that is necessary to win.

Sex

Few would dispute the proposition that, physiologically, an orgasm releases psychic and muscular tension in the body, both leading to good sleep and relaxation. Further psychological benefits would depend very much on the situation. If your experience of physical bonding with another brings a sense of happiness, self-worth, self-esteem, fills your need to bring joy to one another, and makes you feel alive and involved, then that experience plays a role in emotional healing.

Revisit your childhood

Many people did not have an idyllic childhood. Virtually everyone, however, has a few favorite memories from that simpler time. Calling those times back to memory can warm our spirits and put the frustrations of work, parenting, or other matters into perspective. As we discuss in the next chapter, psychologists and psychiatrists recognize that one's childhood is not just a hunting ground for trauma but also for moments of lasting joy.

Summing up for now

There are 168 hours in your week. Let's say that you devote one of those hours, or perhaps even two or three, to medical and mental health appointments. That leaves the vast majority of your time in the charge of just one person: you. What you do with those hours on behalf of your own health will *matter* in the quality of your living and the pace of your recovery from illness.

Barbara... A.P.D., loved ones, and getting help

This segment is perhaps the most painful for me to write. But to be completely honest about my experience with anxiety, panic, and depression, I have to include the difficult story of how A.P.D. affects my marriage and family. I realize that many of you reading this book are not married. However, I suspect that you can relate what I'm going to tell you here to your closest emotional ties, whether with a romantic relationship, with a close friend, or relative.

There is absolutely no aspect of my experience with panic, anxiety, and depression that I haven't shared with my husband, Jim. He has "talked me down" from panic and anxiety more times than I can count. He has seen me at my worst, a trembling, panicky bundle of terror and suffering.

On many calmer occasions, we've talked through what I experienced. He has accompanied me to various doctors and sat in on solemn discussions of breathing exercises, mental gymnastics to forestall panic, tranquilizers, antidepressants, and the rest. He has enthusiastically cheered on any progress I seemed to be making, and gallantly tried to help me deal with my heartbreaking moments when anxiety and panic returned unexpectedly and in full force.

He hasn't shared with me what must be his own conscious or unconscious frustrations from living with an emotional invalid (I have to own up to the reality). He's a good tennis player and would love to have me as a partner for single or mixed doubles. Golf is the same story. He loves being out with his friends on the golf course and there are many occasions when we could both be out there playing with couples we know.

Except for me. I've panicked before on both tennis courts and the golf course. That leaves a major memory scar that can't be wished away. I'm at the point where I'm tired of setting myself up for new embarrassment or relying on my husband to somehow help me gut through something I'm not enjoying.

What's not to enjoy about tennis and golf? I'm increasingly prone to panic when I get hot and out of breath and that comes with the territory in tennis, especially as I get older. And golf courses share all the same fright inducers as do ocean liners or hikes in the forest. I'm at a considerable distance from help or a private safe spot where I can relax, recover from anxiety, and get it back together. If I panic on the sixth hole, you're about half a mile or more away from the clubhouse, the relative security of the restroom as a place to "crash," and access to a phone if this attack somehow turns out to be "the big one."

That supportive role has to wear on him, particularly in his own moments of stress. Although we willingly "carry" the person we love from time to time, it's only natural that we should look forward to some relief from our burden, partly for our own sake and partly for the sake of the suffering person. From the bottom of my heart, I want to spare Jim from his own worry and exertions on my behalf.

Help usually involves getting a referral to a mental health professional from your personal physician. In my experience, this referral process isn't always easy or effective. Some physicians hesitate to turn a patient over to what may be expensive months of therapy once a week or more. Other physicians may feel that their own knowledge of antidepressants, and their ability to prescribe these drugs, makes it unnecessary for the patient to seek another doctor's care.

But let's say your physician does give you a referral to a psychologist or you end up finding one yourself. In my limited experience, psychologists believe that I have been thinking wrong due to past traumas, emotional blocks, or conditioning and need their help in thinking right (including learning to focus, relax, breathe, and so forth). I think they're right. I have been thinking wrong. I'm eager to think right. But there is a very long road between wanting and having.

Or you may be referred to a psychiatrist. In this case you will probably leave the office after the first visit with a prescription for one of the many drug therapies for anxiety, panic, or depression explained in this book. Your contact with the psychiatrist in future weeks and months will consist largely of "checking in" so the psychiatrist can monitor the often-gradual effects of the chosen drug therapy.

In addition, you will be urged to join a therapist-supervised discussion/sharing group made up of people who suffer from anxiety, panic, and depression.

Whether you become involved with a psychologist, psychiatrist, or group, you are fulfilling your spouse's desire for you to get help. It isn't my purpose to make judgments of any form of this help based just on my experience. What I do want to point out is that, for me and probably many A.P.D. sufferers, "getting help" isn't a one-time, one-stop experience. There will be a string of doctors separated by short- or long-term signs of progress in relief of symptoms. "Honey, we've got to get you some help" isn't said once in a marriage, but probably several times. Especially if your first few experiences with mental health professionals are less than productive, you may become increasingly unmotivated to get help.

And money plays a part in this for most of us. Psychologists and psychiatrists are not shy about signing a patient up for what may turn out to be dozens of visits, each at $125 per hour or more. Health insurance will pay for only a limited number of these visits, and then even only a fraction of the cost. Getting help may be more of a gesture of caring than a real suggestion when the family budget just doesn't have an extra $500 or more per month to pay for Mom's therapy.

In addition, your own optimism about professional help may wane. The hopeful desperation that sent you to your first psychologist or psychiatrist may not be sustained as you toddle off to your fourth or fifth, during a period of years. "Honey, we've got to get you some help" may become more and more a refrain of frustration and deep sadness on the part of your spouse rather than a concrete call to action.

10 | What Can a Psychologist, Psychiatrist, Counselor, or Therapist Do for Me?

Patients seeing a physician for anxiety, panic, and depression may also be encouraged by their doctor to develop a trusting relationship with an empathetic psychotherapist. It is true that it is cheaper to talk to a friend, family member, minister, priest, or rabbi, but the advice and evaluation of a talented professional who sees these things every day will give you the confidence that your burdens are not unique and can be lightened. You'll also be relieved from the possible guilt that, for some, accompanies the sharing of your deepest pangs and pains with those you love.

The basic tenet of psychotherapy is not to solve the problem for you, but rather to help you discover the solution for yourself. Many people do not learn how to solve their problems nor to interact successfully with others while growing up. A disruptive household, poor parenting strategies, abuse, and other factors may have gotten in the way of the development of these basic skills.

As a consequence, many enter the adult world not only lacking these skills, but also not knowing that they don't have them. They fail over and over for no reason that they can fathom. Psychotherapy can help them find this reason, and, on occasion, turn their lives around.

Growth requires both insight and then an appropriate response to that insight, which is a change in behavior. If you have insight and are unable to change your behavior, the result can be frustrating. You must enter a relationship with a psychotherapist with the understanding that you may find out things about yourself you have been so far unwilling to recognize or accept. Perhaps the most difficult of all, face the fact that the only response that will lead to healing will be a change in behavior you have been resisting.

Dr. Harold Bloomfield puts the matter well: "To break free of the web of anxiety, you may have to give up a lot. You may have to give up feeling sorry for yourself, straining to be someone you are not, hiding the parts of yourself you fear are unacceptable, and worrying about what others may think. You may have to forgive yourself and others for not being perfect, and stop expecting superhuman feats from others and yourself. You may have to learn to accept parts of yourself that you have resented your entire life. Indeed, you can grow to appreciate yourself exactly as you are and not as you wish you could be."

In choosing a psychotherapist, you may want to get a recommendation from a friend, family member, or your physician. There are many different personal styles of psychotherapeutic practice; your physician can help you match your needs and personality to the psychotherapist best suited to you.

There is no one model for the ideal therapist. In general, it's desirable that he or she is empathetic, has a sense of humor, puts you at ease, is flexible and open, is not condescending, is supportive of your sensibilities regarding treatment options, gives you appropriate feedback and answers your questions, and is willing to see others who may be involved in your illness (such as family members). The most important test, however, is how you feel when you leave their office. Are you more hopeful, feeling you have greater insight, with some plan of action or strategy to include in your daily routine? Are you more empowered with enhanced self-esteem, or still feeling "lost in space"? If you do not feel comfortable with one therapist, try others until you do. This freedom to change is one way in which you take charge of your own dilemma.

Cognitive behavioral therapy

Cognitive behavioral therapy is the most recognized psychotherapeutic approach to treating anxiety disorders, including stress and adjustment disorders (such as posttraumatic stress disorder), generalized anxiety disorder, social and specific phobias, panic disorder, or OCD. It has even proven useful in chronic fatigue syndrome patients.

The purpose of cognitive behavioral therapy (CBT) is to resolve inhibitions, desensitize fears, and increase assertiveness. Its ultimate goal is to allow the patient who has misconceptions and distorted thoughts that contribute to their anxiety to finally see the world accurately. How many of us have the distorted perception that we are the focus of attention, that everyone else is looking at us and thinking critical thoughts about us? That kind of thinking might lead to a lot of anxiety, not to mention paranoia. Listed below are ways that CBT helps with specific problems:

1. **Stress and Adjustment Disorders:** CBT teaches stress reduction techniques, and asks the patient to keep a daily log of stress precipitators: What makes it better, and what makes it worse. It teaches early recognition and removal from a stress source before full-blown symptoms of anxiety occur. The technique of role playing is sometimes used to help teach a new behavior response (such as assertiveness when asking for a raise), which the patient practices over and over until it seems natural.

2. **Social and Specific Phobias:** With another technique called systematic desensitization, the therapist progressively exposes the patient to the stressful stimulus in a controlled environment to gradually relieve the anxiety that is triggered by that stimulus.

3. **Generalized Anxiety, Panic Disorder, and OCD:** With anxiety disorders, the combination of cognitive therapy along with medication is more effective than either alone. A number of behavioral techniques can be used to alter the precipitating factors or secondary rewards that support an anxiety-provoking response. Desensitization by exposing the patient to graded doses of a phobic situation

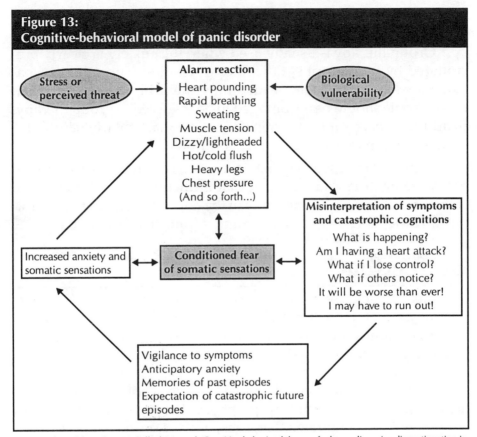

Figure 13:
Cognitive-behavioral model of panic disorder

Source: Adapted from Otto M, Pollack M, et al. Cognitive-behavioral therapy for benzodiazepine discontinuation in panic disorder patients. *Psychopharmacol Bull.* 1992;28:123-130.

is effective and can be practiced by the patient at home as well. A study on OCD by University of California at Los Angeles researchers showed that CBT can actually change the way the brain functions and processes external stimuli. Twelve of 18 patients with OCD studied were found to have different brain scans after treatment compared to before treatment. The change showed up as significantly reduced activity in the caudate nucleus, an area of the brain known to be overactive in OCD.

4. **Chronic Fatigue Syndrome:** CBT was shown to help 70 percent of chronic fatigue patients improve their physical functioning and energy level in a study published in the March 1997 issue of the *American Journal of Psychiatry*.

Group therapy/support groups

Group therapy is usually used when the anxiety is clearly precipitated by the patient's difficulties in dealing with others. If patients are having problems with family members or partners, then these people should be encouraged to be involved in group therapy. In addition, peer support groups have been particularly helpful for patients with panic disorder and agoraphobia.

Support groups for a variety of related conditions, such as alcoholism, gambling addictions, sexual addictions, and violence are active in nearly every community in the country. Most generally follow a 12-step format in a positive and supportive environment.

Biofeedback

Biofeedback uses a variety of sensitive electronic instruments that measure and monitor various changes in the body, such as skin temperature, electrical conductivity of the skin, and muscle tension. These aspects of our physical bodies fluctuate in direct correlation with our brain wave patterns during states of relaxation and stress. State-of-the-art computer technology is used to interpret a range of incoming data from electromyography, galvanic skin response, skin temperature and respiratory feedback, heart rate, and neurofeedback (electroencephalogram).

By observing the feedback on the computer screen, a person can be taught to gain conscious control over brain wave fluctuations involved in the relaxation response. The computer output may be in the form of a flower that grows more brilliant and colorful as you relax, but then diminishes and wilts away if you tense up.

Young children can be taught to relax with a video game-like output that features a man walking through a maze. If the child relaxes, the man will move closer and closer to solving the maze, but if they get nervous, the man will move backwards toward the starting point. The most relaxed kid wins! In essence, biofeedback is just another way to help show a person how to relax and how to meditate. A well-trained person will be able to evoke the relaxation response at will. This ability can give the person a sense of psychological security, the confidence that they will be able to stop an anxious thought or abort a panic attack without waiting for a drug to kick in with sedation effects.

Patients learn to manage their own stress by observing their unconscious patterns of unhealthy reactivity. Physiologically, being able to block the stress response has benefits in preventing the body's alarm system from interrupting normal body homeostasis, and keeps the immune system from failing in response to stress.

Dr. William G. (Bill) Barton, Ph.D., MFCC, is nationally known for his 25 years of work in this field. His program of stress management involves 12 sessions. Each is composed of biofeedback, training for stress and relaxation, monitored relaxation, breathing, and meditation exercises, along with education in cognitive/behavioral stress management. Dr. Barton's philosophy is that "everyone can benefit to some degree from training with biofeedback. Biofeedback and stress management skills assist and encourage the individual in taking some responsibility in his or her own health and well-being."

Guided imagery and visualization

Emotive imagery, in which the patient imagines the anxiety provoking situation while at the same time learning how to relax, is helpful in decreasing anxiety when the situation must be faced in real life. Visualization techniques involve teaching people how to quiet their minds, focus, and use imagery. For instance, this technique has been used very successfully in athletes who wish to better their playing abilities. A golfer may imagine the perfect swing and practice it repeatedly while breathing calmly and learning to relax and focus before hitting the ball.

In an August, 1993 article in the *Practical Horseman,* riding trainer John French describes how he uses visualization to improve the outcome of a class or competition: "Before I go in the ring, I think about how the horse I'm riding feels when he's going really well; I recall a couple of good practice jumps in the ring or a good round we've had in another class."

Laura Carter of Inner Resource Consulting in San Rafael, California, recently explained how she works with athletes in a variety of sports. "I'm currently working with a golfer who has lowered his par from 86 to 76 in three weeks," she said, "and he's now very relaxed on the golf course again and having fun. In his case, it was not a medical problem but a confidence issue." Ms. Carter feels that the techniques she uses to help athletes, including guided imagery, visualization, and hypnotherapy, could also be used on executives to improve anxiety and confidence problems. She has devised a self-hypnosis program that utilizes visualization and can be used in preparation for a stressful event or performance. Here's her formula:

1. Sit comfortably with your arms and legs uncrossed.
2. Take deep breaths and relax slowly from head to toe, feeling waves of relaxation washing over you. Relaxing music may be helpful.
3. Take yourself to the place where you will perform your skill. Notice textures, colors, and movement. Be aware of physical sensations, emotions, and temperatures. Listen for background noises, voices, and your own thoughts. Notice smells.
4. Be an expert. Imagine yourself performing your skill perfectly. Watch yourself be relaxed and focused, concentrating from beginning to end.
5. Imagine that you are in the audience or on the sidelines. As you watch, feel and hear yourself perform again, perfectly.
6. Complete the full activity while feeling successful and satisfied with your performance.
7. Affirm to yourself that you will incorporate the positive effects of your rehearsal into your next performance or practice.
8. Give yourself positive suggestions, enhancing the success and satisfaction of your performance and slowly open your eyes.

You can memorize these steps, make a tape with long pauses between steps, or have a friend or therapist guide you through the process. According to Laura Carter, "With practice, this skill will become second nature to you, and you will be able to quickly rehearse it anytime and any place, giving yourself the extra edge for success."

Hypnotherapy

We recently asked a well-respected hypnotherapist in Marin County to describe the benefits of hypnosis. Barbara Stockwell of the Advanced Hypnotherapy Center in San Anselmo, California, responded by explaining:

> Hypnosis is a proven, fast, and safe method of altering human behavior because it bypasses the critical factor of the conscious, analyzing mind and works with the subconscious mind as the seat of feelings and emotions. It reduces tension and helps normalize the autonomic nervous system. While in this relaxed and pleasant state, the client can more easily let go of inhibitions. With the help of guided imagery, visualization, age regression, direct or indirect suggestions, systematic desensitization, or whatever modality serves him or her best, the patient moves in the direction of personal fulfillment, freedom of personal choice, feeling self-worth and empowerment.

The hypnotic state is the alpha brain wave pattern that is in the 8 to 13 cycles per second range as measured by the electroencephalogram. In the waking state (or beta pattern), reasoning, logic, and decision making are performed. The alpha state is also the rapid eye movement (REM) stage of sleep when we remember our dreams. The alpha state is purported to be the site of suggestibility, learning, creativity, and imagination.

A deeper dream state is the theta pattern, measured at four to seven brain wave cycles per second. Some have suggested that this is the level of our spiritual awareness. The deepest level of sleep is the delta pattern at 0.5 to three cycles per second. No one knows what goes on down there. When falling to sleep, we usually go in succession from beta to alpha to theta and then delta sleep, then we regress backward through theta to alpha, or REM, sleep. In REM sleep, the brain waves speed up to nearly a waking pattern, and the eyes move rapidly from side to side. A normal night's sleep includes four to five cycles of REM and non-REM sleep, with each cycle lasting 90 to 100 minutes. These sleep cycles seem to be especially important in maintaining good energy, stable emotions, and a normal immune system.

Hypnosis is really a form of guided daydreaming, with the ability to make an impact on our waking state by communicating with our mind while in this less inhibited, more creative, and teachable state.

Hypnosis seems particularly successful in the area of phobias and performance anxiety. According to Ms. Stockwell, "All phobias, depending on the willingness of the patient to make changes and the experience of the hypnotist, can either be reduced or eliminated." She often uses age regression (going back in time while under hypnosis) to look for the cause of a phobia and try to desensitize against it. In order to help a patient prepare for a public speaking engagement, she takes them (while under hypnosis) through the experience of preparing for and giving the presentation in front of an audience.

Another benefit of hypnosis that might appeal to the business-person is motivational enhancement. Some people find they can learn more quickly, retain information better, and have a sense of enthusiasm for their work through a series of hypnotherapy sessions. Smoking cessation can often be successfully addressed with only one hypnotherapy session.

Hypnotherapy sessions last 90 minutes and longer. The time is needed by the therapist for establishing rapport with the patient before the hypnotic induction. Patients on antipsychotic drugs are not good candidates for hypnosis, because those drugs can interfere with alpha brain wave patterns.

There are many common misconceptions about hypnotherapy, according to Ms. Stockwell, that deserve to be dispelled:

1. **"I'm too strong minded; I don't think I can be hypnotized."**
   The more intelligent you are and the better you concentrate, the easier it will be for you to go into a deep trance.
2. **"While under hypnosis I will tell things that I do not want to be known by others."**
   Only the information necessary for the desired change will be released from the subconscious mind.
3. **"If an emergency situation were to arise, I would be stuck in a trance."**
   In the case of an unusual emergency situation, you would snap out of hypnosis right away.

4. **"While into hypnosis I might receive suggestions to do things I don't want to do."**
   Hypnosis creates an emotionalized desire to satisfy the suggested behavior, provided that what is suggested harmonizes with your values and belief system.

5. **"Hypnosis is a mysterious, dark, scary state of being."**
   Hypnosis is a natural state of being with an extraordinarily pleasant quality of relaxation.

6. **"I have never been in a state of hypnosis."**
   If you have ever been lost in thought, or so involved in a TV show that you forgot the time, the people around you, and so forth, you have been in a state of hypnosis. This type of hypnotic trance is very common.

Meditation

This vast area of human experience defies brief discussion. We will confine our interest here to the meditation techniques most applicable to anxiety, panic, and depression: breathing, the relaxation response, and transcendental meditation.

Breathing

Like eating and sleeping, we often take breathing for granted, seeing it only as a necessary function, rather than a potential tool to combat anxiety and promote healing. Almost all meditations include deep, relaxed breathing as an integral part of the exercise. Whether it is during yoga exercise or childbirth, conscious breathing can have profound effects on our internal chemistry.

According to Candace Pert, Ph.D., author of *Molecules of Emotion*, "There is a wealth of data showing that changes in the rate and depth of breathing produce changes in the quality and kind of neurotransmitters." In situations of anxiety and fear, we often hold our breath, as if holding in our emotions. At such a time when the brain could use some extra oxygen, it's actually getting less. This is a learned response that, through meditation, we can begin to unlearn.

The first step is to learn how to consciously take just one breath. Find a comfortable sitting position and loosen your clothing if it is too restrictive. Straighten your back, relax your shoulders, and gently close your eyes. Now completely clear your mind to all of your daily problems and responsibilities — let your mind relax and think of nothing. Slowly take a deep breath in, paying attention to how it feels as your chest and lungs fill. Does it feel warm or cool as the air steams into your nose and mouth? Imagine the air drawing the oxygen through your lungs and out into every cell in your body, bringing energy and light to each individual cell.

Hold this breath for a few moments as you imagine the great benefits it is bringing into your body. Then slowly (with back still straight and shoulders relaxed) let the air escape as the lungs naturally recoil and deflate. Let all the tension, stress, and negative thoughts and feelings escape along with the exhaled air. At the end of the exhalation pause for a moment and be thankful for the privilege of being alive, then slowly open your eyes.

You cannot overdose on this relaxation technique, and the more you practice it, the more it works. Soon, you can do it anytime, anywhere for quick resolution of anger, frustration, or anxiety. In fact, a 1994 study by G. Hendricks and K. Hendricks titled "Effects of Daily Breathing on Tiredness and Tension" showed that people who use breathing exercises as part of their daily routine were able to cut their levels of anxiety and stress in half. One might think of this one-breath exercise as the simplest form of meditation, or even a brief prayer.

The relaxation response

Dr. Herbert Benson, M.D., renowned Harvard University research scientist and author of many books, including *The Relaxation Response*, *The Mind/Body Effect*, and *Beyond the Relaxation Response*, has studied and documented the physiologic basis of relaxation and meditation. He and R. Keith Wallace, Ph.D., showed how, through practice of meditation, a person could reduce stress, reduce insomnia, lower blood pressure, control panic attacks, relieve headaches, decrease chest pains caused by coronary artery disease, alleviate anxiety symptoms (such as nausea, vomiting, diarrhea, short temper, and inability to get along with others), and otherwise enhance their physical and mental well-being. These benefits were accompanied by hormonal alterations and increased alpha waves from the cerebral cortex that were consistent and reproducible. Dr. Benson devised a simple technique to elicit the relaxation response in a four-step meditation procedure:

1. Find a quiet environment.
2. Consciously relax the body's muscles.
3. Focus for 10 to 20 minutes on a mental devise, such as the word "one" or a brief prayer, saying the word or prayer with each exhalation.
4. Assume a passive attitude toward intrusive thoughts.

More recently, Dr. Benson has recommended that an individual add to this technique their innermost personal beliefs, which he calls the "Faith Factor," to enhance and deepen the experience of meditation.

An example of a multiperspective therapeutic approach

Dr. Mitchell L. Gaynor, director of medical oncology at Strang Cancer Prevention Center in New York, has devised a group session for patients with cancer. Through a combination of musical sounds and meditation, Dr. Gaynor is able to help the anxious cancer patient move away from a state of fear and reconnect with what is most alive and disease free within themselves. Gaynor's sessions begin with a meditation, accompanied by Gaynor playing "singing bowls," traditional instruments used by Tibetan monks.

The music evokes a sense of the sacred and transports the participants from the conference room to a mountaintop monastery. As patients focus on their breathing, Gaynor guides them by a series of ancient sacred sounds to help them "move inward, to experience an inner silence. The activity is designed to bring the patient beyond the relaxation response to a harmonious state where inner peace is achieved. Before ending the meditation, he reminds patients that they can come back to this place of peace and calm just by working with their breath.

As expressed by Hermann Hesse in *Siddhartha*, "Within you there is a stillness and a sanctuary to which you can retreat at any time and be yourself."

In his book, *Sounds of Healing: A Physician Reveals the Therapeutic Power of Sound* (Broadway Books, 1999), Dr Gaynor tells the story of a patient with metastatic breast cancer who, out of fear and anxiety, refused to have chemotherapy treatment. After participating in the sound meditation therapy, she agreed to the chemotherapy, as well as the recommended bone-marrow transplant. She is now in complete remission from her malignancy. A Bronx woman commented on how the group sessions "...completely relax me. That peaceful feeling lasts for days."

Another patient has said that Gaynor's method has inspired her to make positive life changes that have turned her battle with cancer into "the most beautiful time of my life." Gaynor's unique program is made possible by a growing openness to spiritual and faith-based practices as adjuncts to traditional medical treatment.

Prayer

Even the mention of prayer may set off warning signals for some readers: Do these authors have a particular spirituality or religious perspective to promote? Have I wandered into Sunday School by mistake?

No. These pages don't concern what or if you believe. Nor is it our place here to map out spiritual landscapes for anyone. This being said, however, a discussion of prayer does belong in a book on anxiety, panic, and depression.

No doctor, be him or her theist, atheist, or agnostic, would counsel a patient against the personal choice to involve prayer in recovery from an illness. Why is this? Because prayer, though it may not change things miraculously at times, has a great track record for changing people.

We can interpret this apparent power of prayer as we individually choose. Some will see its power as the result of a redirection of personal problems to some other object or being ("pray to Christ," "pray to the saints," and so forth), the calming effects of sensory deprevation through closed eyes and focused mind, the benefits of the relaxation response, or the subconscious return to a state of dependence and trust on the Deity.

This is the defense of "secular reflection" practiced by many without specific reference to doctrines, God, or a universal spirit. Instead, secular reflection focuses on the deepest yearnings of the heart — "I desperately want my daughter to recover," "I'm afraid of dying," and so forth. These words pass from ourselves to ourselves, like so many other self-dialogues we've had throughout our lives as we talk ourselves in and out of trouble.

For other individuals (and perhaps most of those worldwide who pray), secular reflection isn't prayer at all. These people have deeply held or felt convictions about God, a universal spirit, or a supervising intelligence of some sort whom can be contacted by closing one's eyes and thinking or saying heartfelt words. Any benefits derived from this spiritual or religious form of prayer are interpreted by the faithful as "power from a divine source" for personal renewal. The prayer connection is considered a channel through which spiritual power — and even miracles — flow into individual lives.

The key question for unbelievers, of course, is whether one can reap the psychological benefits of prayer while doubting all along (or completely denying) that any force or presence is contacted or conjured by prayer. Clearly, the answer to that nettlesome problem can only be answered individually. But whatever beliefs you find within, you may want to try prayer. It has no known side effects.

Transcendental Meditation (TM)

Meditation offers an opportunity to get "out of oneself" to other realms of thought and feeling. Various philosophers and theologians have attached names to this "beyond the self" experience. By whatever name, the interconnectedness with others one feels in this space is calming and renewing.

Transcendentalism asserts that, although we may all be very individual and play our own unique tune, underneath is the tone that is the source of all music and all life, constant and forever. It is not necessary that you buy into some theory of the universe to achieve the benefits of Transcendental Meditation (TM).

At root, TM is a practical and easily learned program built on ancient principles and corroborated by modern scientific research.

There are local TM centers listed in the telephone directories of most cities. An introductory lecture is usually offered at no charge. In writing on TM, psychiatrist Dr. Harold H. Bloomfield points out the reason for TM's success in helping those with anxiety disorders: "Meditation elicits a unique state of the body, mind, and spirit that is the exact opposite of stress—a 'stay and play' instead of a 'fight or flight' response."

🐚 A final summing up

You now have before you the panorama of what is involved in the journey through and out of anxiety, panic, and depression. You may have marked your place somewhere on that journey. We hope that these pages will help you see the steps that lie yet ahead.

Despite expert voices on all sides, the voice that matters most in interpreting emotional struggles and setting the agenda for improvement is your own. Take a moment— and right now would be ideal— to listen to what your innermost self thinks and feels. If you listen and hear nothing, be patient. Perhaps your voice has been told to shut up over and over in recent years. Listen until you hear, deeply and intuitively. Then pay attention to the message and act on it in constructive ways.

As you listen to that personal inner voice, we urge you to follow where it leads. For some readers, a medical journey lies ahead, with a trusted physician to support therapy and provide expertise. For others, the journey will be more spiritual in nature, perhaps involving the counsel of a caring religious or spiritual leader. For others, the spiritual journey may be more into the human heart than into the mind of God. Still others will feel good about themselves and others, know that their synaptic clefts are well greased with neurotransmitters, will go on about their business and play. For them, that may be enough—and that's okay.

The point for our purposes is this: Don't let others (including your authors) define this journey for you. *But do take it,* as your best lights guide you. Anxiety, panic, and depression are rumblings of deep tensions, shiftings, and realignments inside. You can prevent a destructive personal earthquake by getting to know those deeper realities — in effect, getting to know (and like) yourself.

We wish you well on the journey. Know that we are on it too.

James C. Gardner, M.D.

Arthur H. Bell, Ph.D.

The final word on *Barbara*:

Although Barbara continues in treatment for her illness, she has made remarkable progress recently through a combination of drug therapy and supportive psychological counseling. In her words, "There are still a lot of clouds in my personal sky, but the sunlight is breaking through more and more often. When it does, it feels wonderful. I'm trying to build on those recurring experiences of peace and joy."

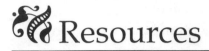 Resources

Reprinted with permission from the August 15, 1999 edition of *Patient Care* magazine

GOVERNMENT AGENCIES

National Institute of Mental Health
6001 Executive Blvd Rm 8184 MSC 9663
Bethesda, MD 20892-9669 (301) 443-8410
www.nimh.nih.gov
Part of the National Institutes of Health, this institute offers public information and conducts research on mental disorders. Links to special sections on both anxiety and depression offer excellent professional information.

Substance Abuse and Mental Health Services Administration
US Dept of Health and Human Services
5600 Fishers Lane Room 15-99
Rockville, MD 20857 (301) 443-0001
www.samhsa.gov
This agency's mission is to improve the quality and availability of services for substance abuse and mental health.

ORGANIZATIONS

Academy of Psychosomatic Medicine
5824 N Magnolia
Chicago, IL 60660 (773) 784-2025
www.apm.org
The organization promotes the practice of consultation-liaison psychiatry and sponsors *Psychosomatics Journal.*

American Academy of Child and Adolescent Psychiatry
3615 Wisconsin Ave, NW
Washington, DC 20016
(202) 966-7300
www.aacap.org
Devoted to understanding developmental, behavioral, emotional, and mental disorders affecting children and adolescents.

American Academy of Clinical Psychiatrists
PO Box 45870
Glastonbury, CT 06033
(860) 633-5045
www.aacp.com
Dedicated to the private practice of psychiatry, this organization has as its goal the advancement of clinical psychiatry.

American Psychiatric Association
1400 K St, NW
Washington, DC 20005 (202) 682-6000
www.psych.org
This internationally recognized society with 42,000 members specializes in the diagnosis and treatment of mental and emotional illnesses and substance disorders, it sponsors the *American Journal of Psychiatry* and *Psychiatric News* publications.

American Psychoanalytic Association
309 E 49th St.
New York, NY 10017
(212) 752-0450
www.apsa.org
A professional organization for psychoanalysts, this association has a hypertext listing on its Web site of members available for referrals.

American Psychological Association
750 First St., NE
Washington, DC 20002
(202) 336-5500
www.apa.org
With 161,000 members, including student affiliates, this is the largest professional organization representing psychologists in the country,

American Psychosomatic Society
6728 Old McLean Village Dr.
McLean, VA 22101
(703) 556-9222
www.psychosomatic.org
This society is a forum for enhancing understanding of how the body and mind interact.

Anxiety Disorders Association of America
11900 Parklawn Dr., Suite 100
Rockville, MD 20852
(301) 231-9350
www.adaa.org
This national, nonprofit organization works to prevent and cure anxiety disorders.

National Alliance for the Mentally Ill
200 N Glebe Rd, Suite 1015
Arlington, VA 22203-3754
(703) 524-7600
www.nami.org
This organization aims to "eradicate mental illness and improve the quality of life of those affected by these diseases." Good source of patient information.

National Depressive and Manic-Depressive Association
730 N Franklin St., Suite 501
Chicago, IL 60610-3526
(800) 826-3632
www.ndmda.org
Educates patients and physicians on depressive and manic-depressive illness. A grassroots network of 275 chapters supports the effort.

National Foundation for Depressive Illness, Inc.
PO Box 2257
New York, NY 101 16
(800) 239-1265
www.depression.org
This organization provides information to physicians and patients about affective disorders.

Society for Neuroscience
11 Dupont Circle, NW Suite 500
Washington, DC 20036 (202) 462-6688
www.sfn.org
Dedicated to understanding the brain, spinal cord, and peripheral nervous system, this organization uses research from medical specialties, including neurology, neurosurgery, psychiatry, and ophthalmology.

BOOKS

The Anxiety Disorders
Noyes R, Hoehn-Saric R. Cambridge, Mass: Cambridge University Press; 1998.

Depression and Physical Illness
Robertson MM, Katona CLE, eds. New York, NY: John Wiley & Sons; 1997.

Diagnostic and Management Guidelines for Mental Disorders in Primary Care: ICD-10 Chapter V Primary Care Version
World Health Organization. Kirkland, Wash: Hogrefe & Huber Publishers; 1997.

Diagnostic and Statistical Manual of Mental Disorders, Fourth Edition
Washington, DC: American Psychiatric Association; 1994.

Diagnostic and Statistical Manual of Mental Disorders, Fourth Edition – Primary Care Version
Washington, DC: American Psychiatric Association; 1995.

Family-oriented Primary Care: A Manual for Medical Providers
McDaniel SH, Campbell TL, Seaburn DB. New York, NY: Springer Publishing Co; 1990.

High-Yield Psychiatry (Science of Review)
Fadem B, Simring SS. Hagerstown, Md: Williams & Wilkins; 1998.
Integrated Primary Care: The Future of Medical and Mental Health Collaboration
Blount A, ed. New York, NY: WW Norton & Co, Inc; 1998.

Managing Mental Health Problems. A Practical Guide for Primary Care
Kates N, Graven M. Kirkland, Wash: Hogrefe & Huber Publishers; 1998.

Mental Disorders in Primary Care
Miranda J, Hohmann AA, Attkisson CC, et al., eds. San Francisco, Calif: Jossey-Bass; 1994.

MGH Guide to Psychiatry in Primary Care
Stem T, Herman J, Slavin P, eds. New York, NY: McGraw Hill Publishing Co; 1997.

Panic Disorder Clinical, Biological, and Treatment Aspects
Asnis GM, van Praag HM, eds. New York, NY: John Wiley & Sons; 1995.

Pocket Handbook of Primary Care Psychiatry
Kaplan M, Sadock BJ. Hagerstown, Md: Lippincott Williams &Wilkins; 1997.

Pocket Handbook of Psychiatric Drug Treatment.
Kaplan HI, Sadock BJ. Hagerstown, Md: Lippincott Williams & Wilkins; 1997.

Pocket Psychiatry
Bhui K, Weich S, Lloyd K. Philadelphia, Pa: WB Saunders & Co; 1996.

Preventing Mental Illness: Mental Health Promotion in Primary Care
Jenkins R, Ustun TB, eds. New York, NY: John Wiley & Sons; 1998.

Primary Care Psychiatry
Knesper DJ, Riba MB, Schwenk TL. Philadelphia, Pa: WB Saunders & Co; 1997.

Primary Care Psychiatry and Behavioral Medicine: Brief Office Treatment and Management Pathways
Feinstein RE, Brewer AA, eds. New York, NY: Springer Publishing Co; 1998.

Psychiatry for Primary Care Physicians
Goldman LS, Wise TN, Brody D, eds. Chicago, Ill: American Medical Association; 1998.

Rapid Psychological Assessment
Olin JT, Keatinge C. New York, NY: John Wiley & Sons; 1998.

Stranger Than Fiction: When Our Minds Betray Us
Feldman MD, Feldman JM, Smith R. Washington, DC: American Psychiatric Press; 1998.

Stress, the Immune System and Psychiatry
Leonard BE, Miller K, eds. New York, NY: John Wiley & Sons; 1995.

Women's Mental Health in Primary Care
Zerbe KJ. Philadelphia, Pa: WB Saunders & Go; 1999.

CLINICAL JOURNALS

American Journal of Geriatric Psychiatry
Journal of Psychotherapy Practice and Research
American Psychiatric Press, Inc.
1400 K St, NW
Washington, DC 20005 (202) 682-6262
www.appi.org

Archives of General Psychiatry (A publication of the American Medical Association)
515 N State St
Chicago, IL 60610
(312) 464-5000
www.ama-assn.org/public/journals/psyc/psychome.htm

Families, Systems & Health: The Journal of Collaborative Family HealthCare
PO Box 20838
Rochester, NY 14602-0838
(716) 244-6050
www.fsh.org

Journal of Clinical Psychiatry: Primary Care Companion to the Journal of Clinical Psychiatry Physicians Postgraduate Press
PO Box 752870
Memphis, TN 38175-2870
(901) 751-3800
www.psychiatrist.com

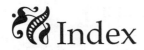 Index